"Moms everywhere, rejoice! *Kids Are Turds* gives you permission to whine into your (much-needed) wine as you flop down in exhaustion after another day of wiping up the unmentionable mess you know will magically reappear tomorrow. Laugh it off, ladies—let Jenny show you how."
—Karen Moline, coauthor of the *New York Times* bestseller, *Sh*tty Mom: The Parenting Guide for the Rest of Us*

"I couldnt wait to review this project, and it did not disappoint. I have been a longtime follower of Jenny's blog and Facebook page and *love* them! Her real talk approach to parenting makes you feel like you're not failing to live up to some unrealistic standard. Even with her blunt honesty you can see her deep love for her children throughout the book. It's a great reminder that we *all* go through times like this, and we're all doing the best we can. Thank you, Jenny, for bringing humor and creativity to this life we call mommyhood!"
—Dawn Recor, blogger of *Diary of a Not So Wimpy Mom*

"Getting shockingly emotional over soup commercials, treating solo grocery-store trips like tropical vacations, staying up and watching kiddie cartoons hours after her kids have gone to bed . . . and, of course, compiling a blackmail album for when her boys get old enough to date? Jenny Schoberl's *Kids Are Turds* is a ridiculously funny and heartfelt chronicle of what it means to be a mother, and whether falling into parental stereotypes is something to fight—or something to embrace with all your heart."
—Dressler Parsons, Student-Tutor.com

Kids Are ~~Turds~~ ~~Terrific~~

Brutally Honest Humor for the Pooped-Out Parent

Jenny Schoberl

author of the *Holdin' Holden blog*

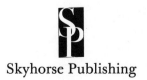

Skyhorse Publishing

Skyhorse Publishing books may be purchased in bulk at special discounts for sales promotion, corporate gifts, fund-raising, or educational purposes. Special editions can also be created to specifications. For details, contact the Special Sales Department, Skyhorse Publishing, 307 West 36th Street, 11th Floor, New York, NY 10018 or info@skyhorsepublishing.com.

Skyhorse® and Skyhorse Publishing® are registered trademarks of Skyhorse Publishing, Inc.®, a Delaware corporation.

Visit our website at www.skyhorsepublishing.com.

10 9 8 7 6 5 4 3 2 1

Library of Congress Cataloging-in-Publication Data is available on file.

Cover design by Sarah Brody

Print ISBN: 978-1-5107-0497-8
Ebook ISBN: 978-1-5107-0498-5

Printed in the United States of America

CONTENTS

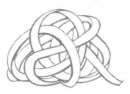

INTRODUCTION

Mom Jeans Anonymous

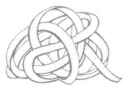

I AM A MOM. THERE. I said it. I don't know why that feels like I'm saying something bad, like I should be speaking in hushed tones in dark alleyways so that no one can hear, but it just feels . . . old. Boring. Frumpy. I am someone's *parent*. The man that I married isn't an eighteen-year-old high school senior anymore; he is someone's *father*. Good ol' Mom and Dad. Yawn.

Day to day, I think being a mom is an awesomely exciting thing, but why does it still feel so strange to say the M-word? Why do I get a full-body shudder whenever I use the word *mom* or refer to myself as a *parent*? I've spent years conducting extensive hands-on, in the field research (a.k.a. blowing 'em out of my crotch and diapering their stinky ends), so I should have answers by now. But I don't. Parenting is just . . . *weird*.

I always thought I would be able to remain the same exact person I was prior to squeezing humans down my pipes and through the trap door. Me? I'm not gonna be a *mom*, I'm gonna be a MILF! I'm gonna drop the baby weight immediately and be so hot with such a killer bod that people will question whether the kids are actually mine. I'll spend the afternoons with my other hot mom friends sipping martinis on the front porch and cackling as we discuss the most scandalous neighborhood gossip. My perfect kids will be at school earning straight A's and will never make any trouble. This whole "parenthood" thing is going to be a piece of cake, and I will be the Sexy Supermom. End of discussion.

I also vowed I'd never be one of those nasally, naggy type moms you see on TV with the school-marm un-styled hair (and definitely *never* the Kate Gosselin infamous porcupine mom-trocity). I'd be the furthest thing from the typical "honey-do" list-making, high-waisted-mom-jeans-wearing, PTA-attending, helicoptering, minivan-driving soccer mom.

The awful word *mom* described those types of women, and that was *not* who I envisioned myself to be. Of course I *knew* I was technically "a mom"; you can't exactly deny that when you have two kids wedged so far up your ass they can smell what you had for lunch yesterday. And let's not forget pain! A body doesn't just forget the torture that is childbirth. Neither does a vagina. Poor vagina.

As much as I loved my kids—and I loved them an embarrassingly huge, going-to-kiss-them-in-public-well-past-their-twenties amount—I never felt like I fell into this "parenthood is my destiny!" groove as easily as everyone else seemed to. I just couldn't ever get into the whole cheerleader mom mindset. No Rah Rah Sis Boom Ba! None of that "I'm Supermom! Being a parent is *so* fabulous! Let's go make crafts out of pinecones!" crap. It actually seemed pretty frickin' obnoxious to me.

And I didn't ever want to be the person who completely handed herself over to her kids. I couldn't become one of those women you see at Walmart who look like they have given up on living their own lives in favor of their children's. The ones who don't even seem to care that they're in public wearing flesh-colored spandex and a dirty, old, too-big t-shirt, or that their kids are screaming bloody murder about wanting a giant box of teeth-rotting cereal. I did *not* want that to be me. I wanted to stay *me*; the *me* that existed before kids got in there and jacked it all up. I could do that, right? I could still be me. My husband, Thomas, and I could still be *us*. With crotchfruit. It was as simple as that. I was pretty sure that I'd just solved Parenthood.

Now, after spawning not one, but two babies, I have the distinct urge to reach back into time and smack the crap out of young me for being such a fucking *idiot*. Way to go, genius! You really called that one. Yes, deary, that was sarcasm. I know it's hard to pick up in your brain's deteriorated state.

So yes, things have most definitely changed. A lot of things. It wasn't until I was intimately familiar with being elbow deep in a diaper change that was more like a Play-Doh fun factory that I realized the truth: no matter how "hip" or "cool" you think you are (and I can't believe I just wrote *hip*. It shows you just how deep into this I really am), once you add children to the pot, your life will never be the same. The progression into accepting parenthood may be one that happens slowly, but my mom always warned me that it *would* inevitably occur. But do we *ever* listen to our parents' advice when we're little? I was positive every bit of wacky advice my mom dispensed was a product of inhaling way too much hairspray from aerosol cans and bleach seeping into her skull. *Obviously* I wasn't going to take her seriously!

But parenthood became my reality, and I learned to accept it. There were many days I spent being unsure if I would *ever* really feel like I'd chosen the right "job," which was a feeling about as annoying as an itchy butthole. Still, I couldn't *make* the job title fit, even if I loved the benefits . . . Y'know, outside of never being allowed to take a sick day.

In an act of sheer desperation (and slight insanity), I decided to start a mommy blog. *Oh, cringe!* I wasn't exactly thrilled about it either, but I needed something to help me not turn into Mommy Dearest, swinging a metal hanger by the end of the day. Something that couldn't interrupt me with things like logic, or reason. In that moment, I swore to myself that I wouldn't be regurgitating fluffy bunnies, rainbows, and bullshit about how my perfect spawn could recite the alphabet backwards and crap in a tiny plastic toilet. If I was going to do this, it had to be *real*. Maybe I'd even find some other moms out there who could relate?

This not-so mom-ish mommy blog turned out to be liberating! Magical! Therapeutic, even. I was finally able to unleash my true thoughts and feelings as a woman who would *never* be taking home a Mom of the Year award. And it definitely helped to keep me from running away with the traveling circus. (Although I was still convinced that I could be the bearded lady in the sideshow. Especially since the kids never give me the time to wax the 'stache.)

Still, blog therapy aside, there were some stories I just couldn't bring myself to write. In my tired brain, they made me less of a mom, or more of a craptastic one. They were too disgusting, disturbing, embarrassing, and/or completely ridiculous. I could write about crapping my pants in public at twenty-one years old, but I couldn't type the words "I just realized there was a giant booger on my shirt all day long. This booger doesn't belong to me. This booger is now a fashion statement."

With this book, it's time to finally tell those stories. Because it sucks balls to feel like you're alone or like you're "not mom enough." The truth is, these disgusting and ridiculous stories—these moments where we find ourselves hiding in the bathroom to eat so we don't have to share our beloved snacks—these are our defining moments. Bet you never thought yanking a turd the size of a Buick out of your kid's butt would be a moment you would look back fondly on, but it is. And that? *That* is being a mom.

CHAPTER 1

A IS FOR A-HOLE, B IS FOR BIG FAT BABY

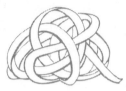

WITH HOW FRIGHTENINGLY POPULAR *TEEN MOM* has become, you might be surprised that at twenty-two years old (or was it twenty-three? Who can remember these things anymore?), Thomas and I were the first among our circles of friends to bring forth new life to this planet. First it was Holden, and then, by complete surprise, came Parker. I still swear he was conceived by Immaculate Conception.

It's not like my friends were all that supportive or under-standing, but Thomas's friends quite literally disappeared from his life. It was like they fell off the face of the earth, or we had unknowingly joined a leper colony or contracted the bubonic plague. Those pesky rats. Or in this case, those pesky sperm. Not knowing any other parents to talk to about kids, it felt like we were flying by the seat of our pants. We had no idea what was "right," or what other parents were doing, or how we should be acting. Completely clueless, party of two!

Now, with a little experience under my belt, I can say that *all* of child-rearing (and why do we call it "rearing"? It isn't as if we give birth from our asses) is nothing but a big, obnoxious, frustrating guessing game. Back then we thought there was some kind of rhyme or reason to everything, but now we know that parenting has no logic. Not a fucking speck of logic in the whole thing.

Every day was a new day of figuring out something a small child could clearly see, but we spent *hours* struggling with. The first few years were like trying to put together an Ikea bed without any instructions; it's fabulous when you *finally* get something into place, but then the whole damn thing falls apart again. Really, we just needed help. And more than anything, I wanted someone who could tell me if all the seeds in my kid's crap were normal, or if my diaper pail was going to start sprouting poop-trees.

It wasn't until sometime *after* I'd survived childbirth for a second time that we caught wind that a friend of Thomas's named Jasmine had just moved back to our area. A very *pregnant* friend of his. And even better—she wanted to get together after she delivered. I won't pretend that four straight years of being shunned hadn't turned me into a bit of a shut-in, but getting out of the house and conversing with someone who had yet to be brain-sucked by the PTA or crazy Pinterest pod people? I jumped at the chance faster than my uterus jumps into oncoming traffic when anyone mentions having another baby.

This get-together just so happened to be her birthday dinner (and I must say, what better birthday present than not being pregnant?), which meant a ton of strangers would be there. But I'd already promised myself a dinner that I didn't have to cook, so there was no backing out. I had never met this friend of Thomas's before; hell, I don't even know how *he* knew her. She could have been a former lover or a mistress, and her brand new fresh from the uterus baby could have belonged to him and I wouldn't have cared. I would have hung out with my smothering mother-in-law to get out of the house. (Okay, no, the hell I would, but trust me when I say the situation was becoming that dire!)

So, of course, we hit it off right away. It was easy to find something in common, being that she'd just propelled a

2

child out of her vagina and I had done that same thing twice before. But this was *more*. I could tell we would be instant friends. We could have talked about anything: movies, music, the giant human-swallowing puddles in the parking lot that nearly killed us all. But yet, the conversation always turned back to *one* subject: kids. Always. We were two young, vibrant women with strong personalities. Confident and mature adults with adult thoughts and opinions on all kinds of worldly subjects, but we just couldn't manage to talk about anything other than our kids.

There we were, seated at the longest table known to man, munching tortilla chips covered in a weird delicious white sauce that I could swear was some kind of ranch, but probably wasn't. (Sometimes it's best not to think too much about these kinds of things.) On every side of us sat her friends—whom I did not know and had never seen before in my life—all there to celebrate the anniversary of the day her face rubbed against her mother's vagina. This was meant to be a festive event, and it was, but we may have killed the mood by casually discussing nipples, bottles, diaper sizes, teething, potty training, sleeping through the night . . . You name the inappropriate child-related subject, and we talked about it. We were in a *zone*.

We were aware of all the other people at the table, but you can bet your sweet ass we didn't pay attention to any of them. But there was one dude who kept shifting uncomfortably in his seat. Every time the conversation happened to turn back to children, he would shift around again. It was distracting as hell! I got enough of that junk at home whenever I tried to do anything relatively important; it was like the kids automatically knew when I needed them to *just be quiet for one second!* and they went into Metallica Mode. It's why I stopped taking phone calls. Soon enough, the man was also breathing heavily from his nose and furrowing his brow. I guess my years as a mom *did* have one perk: the keen ability to sense attitude and douchebaggery from a mile away. I guess spending time with no one but nonsense-spewing children all day and honing my "craft" was finally paying off! I had *kinda* hoped any perks would go to my boobs, but I had quickly learned to take what I could get.

As my brand new BFF (or maybe I should call her my OAF: Only Adult Friend!) Jasmine and I continued yammering about the fruit of our looms, he began to look like one of those freaky, plastic stress relieving heads that resemble a tiny Ross Perot. The ones that, when you squeeze them, the eyes pop out. It was truly a sight to behold. I was mentally taking bets on how much longer he would last before his head just popped right the fuck off.

You might think that, out of respect, we would stop our kid talk, but I do enough coddling of children at home, so there would be no intelligent political banter for him. I couldn't help it; finally having another mother to talk to just felt too natural and relieving. Too bad, so sad for grumpy pants.

By the end of dinner, after two straight hours of eye rolling, heavy sighs, and mumbling under his breath, I guess Mr. Friendly decided he'd had *enough.* He was almost home free, just moments from getting in his car, driving away, and never having to hear about chunky milk vomit ever again. Unfortunately for him, he just couldn't contain his baby rage any longer. We'd just rounded back to discussing diaper changes when he threw his arms in the air and huffed heavily.

"Again? Can't we talk about *anything* else?!" he shrieked.

Both Jasmine and I glanced over at him. I could swear he was foaming from the mouth. As if we were on the exact same wavelength, we replied no. simultaneously and went right back to diaper talk.

Once I became a parent, it became impossible for me to get through a conversation, no matter how short, without bringing up my kids. What the hell is wrong with me? I could be talking to a stranger at a gas station about jet fuel (I have no idea why this would happen, just go with me), and how I thought my house wasn't in any kind of fly zone until a jet flew over our house and—here it comes—woke my kid from a nap. There you have it; from zero to baby in two point five seconds.

But can you guess where foamy-mouthed BabyHater is now? What ever became of such a man? Did he find himself in a county lockup for lashing out at a group of nuns? Did he trap a woman in a well and lower baskets of lotion down to her while dancing around in a suit made from human skin? Did he join a monastery to live a life of peace and solitude away from parents and their small whiny children?

No. None of those. Not even close. He is preparing for the birth of his first child. *And* he plans to be the stay-at-home parent. *And* he can't shut the fuck up about it.

I just hope he feels like a mega-turd for being such a mega-turd.

CHAPTER 2

WHO NEEDS THE BAHAMAS WHEN WE HAVE TARGET?

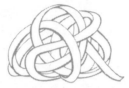

IT'S A LITTLE EMBARRASSING TO admit how long it took me to actually grow a pair of lady-balls and take out both of my kids by myself. I'm still not sure I'm ready to reveal just how lengthy, but know that it was a nonsensically dumb amount of time. Why? Horror stories. Not just losing one of the little boogers, but the knowledge that they are very aware when they outnumber you and use it as a weapon of mass destruction.

Alas, kids insist on being fed every day. When I finally took this huge step (mostly because I thought I would burn the house down if I had to stay in it any longer), I immediately knew I'd made a terrible mistake. Shopping with two kids and no other parent present is a great way to kick your confidence right in the junk. And as much as I love food, I find nothing even remotely enjoyable about the grocery store. Trying to find the best prices with the multitude of coupons I have frustrates me. (What? Coupons rule!) Plus, the cold sections nearly give me hypothermia, and I get some serious road rage pushing my cart down aisles.

I love elderly people and their sweet little voices, orthopedic shoes, and high-watered pants, but being stuck behind them in the soup aisle because they insist on taking up the whole fucking thing and either can't hear you say "excuse me," or simply don't care that you're waiting patiently, makes me wanna ram them in the backs of their heels. Don't act like you got nowhere to be! Knees to chest, granny! Knees. To. Chest!

Thanks to kids and their evil maniacal ways, I developed anxiety just *thinking* about the weekly stock-up trip. I spent far too long trying to justify to Thomas that it was fine to live off of ramen and peanut butter. We don't need milk or bread! I'll just MacGyver the sad contents of our pantry! The store isn't necessary! We'll buy a cow and produce our own milk!

Going to the grocery store with two kids under the age of four should be considered an Olympic sport. Or a new form of torture. They both want to sit in the cart, but in the front. No, wait! The front is uncomfortable—let's both sit in the back! He's taking up all the room! Now he's kicking me! I want out! I want to walk! I have to pee! My legs are tired, put me back in! I want Cocoa Puffs, why can't I have Cocoa Puffs? I never get *anything* I want! No! I don't want that! It's nasty! I don't care if I've never had it, it tastes like vomit!

That is what happens every single time, without fail.

Just send a crime suspect to the store with my two bratty kids (which, let's face it, is all of them); I guarantee they'll squeal in five minutes flat. What should only be a ten-minute "quickie" trip always turns into a forty-five minute whore of a marathon when kids are involved. I only get half of my list and need a nap immediately afterward. Or a strong drink. Or a mallet to the head.

If you're looking for an effective diet—something that will make you naturally detest food—a cart full of children is the solution. Nothing will make you lose your appetite quite like having one kid farting on your apples and bananas, and another one rubbing their entire frickin' body all over the dirty, grimy, grocery store floor like it's a damn

Slip N' Slide and then getting handsy with the rest of the produce. It makes me want to never step foot in a place that sells food again. At least, not with little humanoids (though I'm still not fully convinced we're from the same planet). These horrific outings showed me why the saying "Raising kids is like being pecked to death by chickens" exists. They made me want to scream, but I tried my best to keep my cool. Plus, I didn't have money for bail if I had the breakdown I so deserved right there between the Cheerios and the Cocoa Puffs.

I didn't have the opportunity to experience grocery shopping by myself for many years. By then, my hatred of the grocery store and slow ass grannies in Hoverounds was so violent that I could actually hear my insides sizzling. It almost made me wish this were the sixties and you could light up a smoke right there in the middle of the aisle 7 just to de-stress. Sixties moms always looked so relaxed in pictures . . .

Then one day, something *magical* happened. The stars aligned, the husband came home, and I busted my ass out of the damn house like it was a prison break. Grocery store, ahoy! Without kids! At first, I proceeded with caution. Without the kids along to yank shit off shelves or beg for boxed macaroni and cheese, I wasn't sure what to do with myself. Lo and behold, I *actually* got to casually peruse the aisles, reading labels and checking off my list, instead of white-knuckling the cart and throwing in junk that was close enough to what we needed while grumbling "I fucking *hate* grocery shopping" through my teeth.

It was a rejuvenating experience. For the first time ever, I was happily stuck behind a Hoveround granny instead of wanting to unleash ten years of suppressed road rage. "Take your time! No rush!" I was the Julie Andrews of the grocery store, twirling through the aisles like they were the Swiss Alps. As happy and relaxed as this short break was,

I still thought about the kids the entire time. Even though I'd temporarily escaped their clutches, I could never *really* get away. This was all part of their plan to break me—I was sure of it! I returned home much later (yes, I could have been done in ten minutes, but I took my sweet ass time) feeling more relaxed than that one time my family went to the playground without me.

That day I had a breakthrough: who the hell needs the Bahamas? Going to the grocery store alone is like taking a tropical vacation! Slow ass grannies in moto-scooters? They're just like hot cabana boys hand-feeding you grapes. This must be something only parents understand, because I've gotten a lot of crazy looks when I brag to non-parent friends about how fun it was to go to the doctor without taking the boys with me—even though I was there to get jabbed with needles. A break is a break! And some days, even a root canal sounds appealing.

CHAPTER 3

IF I CALL DINNER "DIN-DIN" ONE MORE TIME, PLEASE PUNCH ME IN THE UTERUS

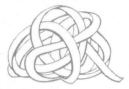

PUBLIC SPEAKING HAS *NEVER* BEEN one of my strong points. In school, I would have full-blown poop attacks any time I had to give an oral presentation in class. Unfortunately, "The Girl with the Vomiting Rectum" was not what I wanted as the byline of my senior portrait. Yet any time I had to stand in front of a room full of people and speak, I would feel my face burning up, that oh-so familiar butt-sick feeling would wash over me, and I'm told (much to my embarrassment) that my nostrils would flare like a fucking horse. And my palms were so clammy on those days that they could have sprouted mushrooms.

Any time I overheard someone say that taking a public speaking class was an "Easy A," I wanted to punt them straight in the no-no bits. What a bunch of liars. There are some things you're born with or you're not; like a love of beets, common sense, and the ability to comfortably speak in front of a group of people without collapsing or wanting to excrete. From your mouth or rear-end. If you got me around a group of my friends, though, all walls were down and the gloves were off. I often compare it to Dr. Jekyll and Mr. Hyde. One moment I was dry heaving and nostril flaring, and the next I was yelling "Son of a Shit-dick-asshole!" in the hallway. Detention was fun!

As I got older and less needy for the approval of my peers, the urge to butt puke became less frequent, as did the requirement to speak in front of groups. No matter how much time passed, though, I still didn't like that nonsense. I am a writer and not a stand-up comedian; it will never be my "thing." One thing I *did* pride myself on was having awesome conversational skills. I had a great vocabulary, detailed and precise stories, and I was known to be a fantastic listener. I'm quite the catch, if I do say so myself. I know, I sound like I'm bragging, and maybe I am. But mostly it's because I admire the person I once was. Having kids changed that faster than I can change a diaper filled with solid shit. (If it's runny, all bets are off.)

It was never in the original "plan" for me to be a stay-at-home mom. Thomas and I never even discussed it. I'd been working full time since I was eighteen, so it was only natural to return once I'd popped some baby goodness all over the place. I liked having an income and being able to contribute to bills and being a productive member of society, but when the time finally came, I just couldn't go back. I couldn't detach myself enough from this squishy little potato-looking thing that had come out of me not long ago. I have zero regrets, but fact is fact! Going from chatting with peers on a daily basis, to 99.9 percent of your conversations being with a tiny baby that does nothing other than scream and shit itself can do a number on your poor tired brain.

For a while, I pretended Holden's grunts and explosive fart faces were responses to the conversations I would try to have just to break the "silence." (And by silence, I mean the lack of real words. There is never *real* silence with a baby in the house.) But I'm not really sure if that helped to keep my skills sharp, or if it only succeeded in making them worse. As much as baby-talk makes me want to go on a stabbing spree with a spork, that shit just happens when

11

you have no access to *real* conversation. Like the clap, baby-talk is a disease, and it likely killed more of my poor brain cells than the red-faced squeezing of two kids down my birth canal did.

As much as I absolutely loved being a stay-at-home mom (which I'll admit has a lot to do with *hating* my days in the workforce), I actually found myself jealous of Thomas when he left to go to work every day. Not just because he got, what to seemed to me, like a break from baby-duty, but also because he got to talk to humans who responded in ways that weren't belching up formula, bloody murder shrieks from the depths of hell, or disgustingly disturbing combinations of the two.

At the end of every week, he looked so put together and well-adjusted, and I, like my kids, was a babbling drool-jockey. And people say lobotomies don't happen in these modern times! Being confined with small children all day every day is kind of like crawling under a rock and staying there for twenty years. You have no idea how far removed from reality you have become until, one day, you leave your gilded mom cage, realize that acid wash is no longer in style, scream "What sorcery is this?!" and fall to the ground in a sobbing heap, crushed by the realization the world has changed and left your ass behind in the dark ages.

That's what happened to me, anyway.

My children would be pleased as punch to know they have made me their bitch. Even when I'm in a crowd of people I have known twice as long as my spawn, I still feel totally awkward and out of place. What do I say? What do I do? I don't have any interesting gossip, and I doubt these people would find a story about how my kid produced a turd nearly as big as his entire body as amusing as I do. What about the promise I'd made to *stay me*? That went out the window along with my skinny jeans.

I guess I should just be thankful that I haven't accidentally started baby-talking grown adults. It doesn't matter that I've adamantly refused to baby talk my kids, because I still fear doing it to others. The brain after children is mysterious—cruel and mysterious. I was always worried of slipping up and having someone say "Um, your 'mom' is showing. You might wanna tuck that back in," and *bam*! Pigeonholed! Back under that rock I would have to crawl. It was time to accept that the chances of holding an intelligent conversation without nearly hurting myself was about as likely as a two-year-old adequately wiping their own ass after an ugly spell of sting-ring.

See? There I go again! All hope is lost.

CHAPTER 4

MINE IS A 4-LETTER WORD

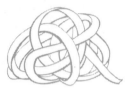

I REMEMBER THE DAYS WHEN I would go to the pantry to get myself a snack, grab a drink from the fridge, and plop my ass on the couch to indulge in the goodies that were all for me and me alone. I felt comfort in knowing that what I had was *all mine* and no one else's. If I wanted to quadruple dip? So be it. If I wanted to make a total slobbery mess of myself? Done. No problem! If someone else wanted a snack? Go get it yourself! You're not helpless!

Sip, munch, sip, munch; those were the days!

I won't beat around the bush here: I didn't know jack *shit* about parenting going into it. How small to cut up food pieces so the kid won't choke? No idea. That washable markers are, in fact, *not* washable? Learned that one the hard way. But one thing I *did* know was that my spawn were going to learn to share. No way in hell was I going to have the shitty little brat standing in the center of a room surrounded by other kids, clutching onto some stupid toy for dear life while screeching "mine!" To most, that word may not be filthy, but to me, it sure as hell falls into the category of Four-letter Words You Don't Want to Hear Escape Your Child's Mouth. I'd honestly rather hear my kids say "Fuck!" than "Mine!" The word is just *that* obnoxious to me.

14

Raising a kid to be a spoiled rotten brat was positively out of the question. To prevent this, I decided to make *sharing is caring* my most uttered phrase. Well, after the word *no*, of course. In a show of solidarity (and so they could never call me a hypocrite once they got past one-syllable words), the sharing in our home extended to adults, as well. Share all the things! With all the people!

It was never difficult to get Holden to share, as he was a very mellow only child for his first two years of life. He never had anyone to play tug-o-war with over a plastic stethoscope or to screech at over who would play with the stupid Matchbox car first. Whenever he found himself around other children, he was probably so excited to interact that he didn't give a floating fart in space about toys getting snatched out of his hands. On many occasions, I would watch him happily relinquish whatever he was playing with to anyone who asked . . . or didn't. Usually didn't. Three cheers for the king of sharing!

Everything changed when Parker was born. I'm not saying the kid ruined Holden's easygoing nature, but the dynamic of siblings is a far cry from that of an only child. Holden was all about sharing with Parker, but Parker was *not* interested in sharing back. Babies must be born as little warriors with the "I must fight for what is mine! It's Battle Royale time, bitch!" mentality. That kid became the awful shithead in the middle of the room holding on to an action figure that doesn't even have a frickin' head while Holden screeched, "Share! You have to share!" Parker was only a year old, and he apparently didn't understand how not to be a brat yet. We had to start all over again with him.

In the beginning, it was like being a prison guard. For some reason, Parker thought that if he didn't defend what was in his hands at all times, it would be stolen by his fellow inmate. Actually, now that I think about it, it didn't really matter whether it was in Parker's hands. If Parker had ever even just *touched* it, Holden could not have it. It was World War Toddler up in that bitch.

To nip this in the bud, we originally tried the method of buying two of everything; they can't possibly fight over shit if we have two of everything! Fail. I decided to set a good example—being that I am the mother and all—by showing my angry, stingy, butt-headed baby that sharing is awesome. Everyone shares! Sharing is great! Do you want some of my water? I'm happy to *share* it with you! Look! Daddy and I are *sharing* this dessert—do you want some? Allow me to *share* it with you!

On our path to a less slap-fighting "mine!"-filled household, the plan took a sharp left turn and backfired on us. Sure, the kids were sharing a little better, but nothing belonged to any one person anymore. This included, but was not limited to, beds, snacks, napkins, and beverage glasses. Sure, sharing is awesome and fantastic. But I'll tell you what is *never* awesome or fantastic: being handed a cracker by your child (who is smiling ever-so-sweetly, which convinces you that all your nagging hard work to instill good values into your precious, innocent little child has *finally* worked) then putting the cracker into your mouth, and only *then* realizing that it has been in their mouth first. That sucker is good and saturated. Excuse me while I vomit. This is the closest to a classic TV spit-take I have ever come. They couldn't just take a bite of the damn thing—*noooooo*, that would be too obvious! My children preferred to lick off all of the salt and then decide they no longer wanted it. "Well, Mommy always said 'sharing is caring!'"

The hardest thing to admit is that I have fallen for this trick more than once. I have wanted to take a windshield scraper to my tongue way too many times to remove the already soggy goo of pre-licked cracker. You would think I'd have learned my lesson by now. But the truth is, I'm stuck. If I so much as hint that they should stop sharing their nasty leftovers, those *years* of nagging will all be in vain.

This sharing madness got to the point where I would have to inspect my drinking glass in search of what I like to call "mouth floaties" before I could take a sip. Backwash, how I loathe thee! I loved that my kids enjoyed a tall glass of water as opposed to soda or any other junk packed with sugar, but I had *zero* interest in choking down the leftover food that was stuck in their creepy little toddler teeth.

Notice the last paragraph was written in past tense, as in I *used* to check crackers for spit, drinks for mouth floaties, and napkins for boogers. Truthfully, it got exhausting to do that with every single damn thing I considered using or consuming every single day of my life. So I just . . . stopped. Yes, it's disgusting and mentally disturbing. Yes, it's unsanitary, and frankly, just lazy. Maybe I should hang my head at how far I've fallen, but I know this to be true: we've all done it at *least* once, haven't we? Humor me. I can't handle the truth right now. I mean . . . their spit is technically *my* spit, so what's the harm?

Don't answer that. Just leave me to my delusions.

CHAPTER 5

THE TALE OF CHICKEN DOODOO, AND WHY MOMS CAN'T FART

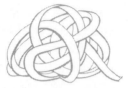

THE FIRST TIME I WAS truly, physically repulsed by Holden was when he was about three years old. I will never forget it. I've tried—trust me. Three years might seem like a long time considering all children are positively disgusting and begin grossing out the world on Day One. That's just a fact of life. Yes, I spent many a diaper change with a shirt wrapped around my face to act as a stench barrier and dry heaving because I swore the poo smelled so bad I could taste it. But to *really* repulse me takes effort. And my boys were up for the challenge.

It was a dark and stormy night; the lights were flickering, and the wind was howling around the house. Okay, okay, I'm joking. It was a completely normal day. One moment, Holden and I were sitting on the couch watching TV, and the next, he had vanished. It wasn't like him to disappear without a sound, so I knew something was wrong. Then I heard a voice call me from the bathroom. Being that I was alone in the house with the boys, and Parker was just a tiny baby who had only mastered the art of screaming, I knew it had to be Holden. Perhaps it was my increasingly old age or the constant ringing in my ears from said screaming baby, but Holden sounded alarmed. And when you hear an alarmed voice calling to you from a bathroom, your ass had better *run* because there's a high probability that your cell phone has taken a nose dive into a toilet full of piss. (Let me tell you that while a pee-soaked phone *may* work again, you will never feel quite the same about holding it up to your face.)

I dashed from the kitchen to the bathroom, but I halted at the doorway when I saw Holden peering into the toilet.

"What? What's wrong? What happened? Are you bleeding? Are you hurt? *What???*"

He looked up at me, an odd glint in his eyes.

"It's a chicken doodoo" he said, pointing toward the bowl.

"A . . . what?"

"A chicken doodoo! It looks like a chicken!"

Obviously, I *had* to look.

I walked up to the toilet and peered down into it, just like Holden had been doing. I did not see a chicken. No, not at all. I saw shit. A giant, disgusting toddler shit. I bent down to get a closer look, willing my brain to figure out how it might possibly, *somehow,* resemble a chicken. And as I came within inches of the toilet bowl, I caught a huge whiff of steaming fresh shit stench. I gagged violently into the toilet and I got a strange feeling in the pit of my stomach. No, not the urge to vomit, but a grisly realization. It wasn't just shit I smelled; it was conspiracy!

And there I was, a grown woman, sitting on a bathroom floor, having just inspected a poop because a toddler told me to do it. It was the first time I was completely and totally repulsed by my own flesh and blood. And Holden loved it. From that moment on, for an *entire* year, Holden named and categorized every single poop that came out of him. His poops could look like animal, object, food—nothing was sacred, and all of it made me want to barf. To top it all off, he took pride in every reaction of barfy repulsion that I had. He delighted in making me squirm and absolutely loved that he could torture me this way. That year, I learned that my sweet toddler was in fact a hardened terrorist with a fondness for fecal torture.

Even worse, Holden was not satisfied with just being nasty himself. It didn't take long for him to get a little brother equally as disgusting as he was, and together, they became a stinky duo of dry heaves and SBDs. These boys—the ones whose diapers I changed for nearly two years a piece, and who still call me for bathroom assistance because even though they can take apart and put back together toy robots, they still can't manage to wipe their own asses—these are the boys who made it their mission to be as repulsive to me as possible. They're the same boys who, for reasons unknown to me, smell like gym socks and burnt hair, pick their noses, and *eat* their toenails with not a care in the world. These boys are the exact same children who have crapped their pants, not told anyone, and then proceeded to hide the offending turd in their closets, forcing me to play a rousing round of Find That Smell. These boys let the dog lick the insides of their mouths, even after I remind them that the dog licks his own poop chute. Ugh. *Those* boys, the loves of my life, fruit of my loins, blossoms of my crotch, they are the most disgusting people I have ever known in my time here on earth.

And that's saying a lot, because I grew up with only an older brother. One who would hold me down, sit on my head, and fart directly into my mouth. I was not *completely* unaware of what I was getting myself into, but I had no idea the eyes of a mother see far more horrific things than that of a sister. It would not surprise me at all if one day I found out my brother played a secret game of Find That Smell with my mom and never told me. Or anyone. After all, I never would have let him live it down.

Even though my lady parts had done me wrong numerous times in my life, it was still tough being the lone vagina in the house. (This is much like being the Lone Ranger. I should procure it a hat. Do they make hats for vaginas?). Finally, I felt the need to put my foot down on the nasty ass shenanigans taking place or be forever lost to the ways of the peen. Not that I'm dainty, but damnit, I *am* a woman, and we have certain standards! For instance, not living in filth or tearing ass at the dinner table while people are still eating. I don't ask for much. Even Thomas, the king of massive bodily functions, was finding himself grossed out on a daily basis by these two little hellions. So one day, we declared that the dinner table would be our nastiness-free zone, where we could have just a few minutes a day of poop-free family time. Things were going great, until one fateful night. We were eating happily, and in the one split second of silence during the whole meal, I accidentally let the *tiniest* toot go from my rear end. It was like the world had stopped spinning.

"Ugh, Mommy! You are *so* gross!" they screeched. They started wailing and holding their noses. Even Thomas looked at me with disgust in his eyes.

Because, obviously, girls don't fart. Especially not girls who are *moms*! It didn't matter that the kids came out of my vag covered in my insides—suddenly, *I* was the nastiest one in the house. All three of them ganged up on me, always ready to catch me doing something gross.

Things went from bad to worse. One day, I slipped up, and they happened to peek in the toilet when I was on my period. Suddenly I wasn't their beloved Mommy anymore—I was an oozing, bloody zombie monster. If I *never* in my life get asked why I have "bloody doodoos" again, it will be too soon.

And just like that, with one solitary toot and one tampon, I was forever branded The Gross One. I could have wallowed in despair about what had become of my life. I could have spent hours whining about how chicken poops and dinner farts were different from my visions of quiet afternoons on the front porch sipping martinis. But instead, I decided to spend those bitter hours plotting my revenge. As much as I believe that bitching is good for the soul, I chose sweet, wonderful payback. Payback in the form of pure blackmail. Six years ago, since Holden came screaming into this world, I began taking photos of Holden and Parker (once he was born) being gross and collecting them in a photo album. Now, that one album has turned into a nice, round forty or so albums, primed and ready to be shown to all future girlfriends. And with every "Ew, Mommy!" I add one more picture.

CHAPTER **6**

HOW TO MANIPULATE YOUR KIDS INTO RELIVING YOUR CHILDHOOD

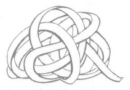

WHEN THOMAS AND I PLANNED our second family vacation to Disney World, we got the idea that we wanted to be like all the sappy commercials and make it a surprise for the kids, who were four and two years old at the time. We were master-minding geniuses, I tell ya! The only problem with this plan was that we'd be driving the entire way to Disney. That's thirteen hours and ~~forty-five thousand~~ twenty-three minutes, to be exact. Overnight. But we knew we had to keep it a secret, or we'd be dooming ourselves to over-excited children who would give up sleeping in favor of whining and hours of chanting "Are we there yet?" That was *not* going to fly.

Our plan was to tell the kids we were going on a "special vacation," but not tell them the destination. Then they would sleep the whole time and wake up just as we were pulling into our resort and bam! Shock! Surprise! Best parents ever! Happiest kids on earth at the happiest *place* on earth!? It was absolutely foolproof. What could possibly go wrong? Do you feel an impending sense of doom? I didn't then, but I do now. Hindsight is a real bitch.

For months, we planned this trip in secret. Any time the kids would see a picture of Disney on the computer screen, I'd quickly make up a ridiculous excuse to explain it away.

Ages four and two may be hellion ages, but they sure are gullible. All of my spare time (well, any rare minutes when they weren't climbing on me like a jungle gym) was spent scheduling, choosing, and planning this vacation down to the very last detail. Where we would eat, what rides we'd go on, what order we'd try to ride them in—everything was planned. *Obsessed* is too mild of a word. I wanted this to be *perfect*. And I was so damned excited, I could hardly contain myself, and I actually found it hard to keep the secret from the boys . . . even though they weren't even asking.

In my mind, I pictured pulling in to the parking lot of the resort, announcing to the kids that the "surprise vacation" was actually Disney World, and them absolutely losing their shit. Screaming, jumping up and down, crying, foaming at the mouth, even a little pants peeing would be a welcome reaction. I wanted full-body freak outs worthy of *America's Funniest Home Videos*. I myself was feeling ready to do all those things, so of course they would be, too.

Almost every summer growing up, my whole family would go to Disney World. All I can cognitively remember from the yearly trips is screaming my face off upon being forced by my mother to ride Space Mountain and being absolutely terrified of cardboard cutouts of witches for no damn reason whatsoever. Somehow, neither of those memories outweighed the joy and anticipation I always had at the end of every school year, knowing a trip to Disney was imminent. So, personally, I could not *wait* to go to Disney again. Honestly, I would live there if I could. In the castle, of course—where else? And judging by the excitement from the boys every time a commercial for the land of the giant rat came on TV, I was fairly confident there would be a moderate amount of pants-wetting going on once the truth was finally revealed. You know you have problems when you've got your fingers crossed for a pee accident.

If I said that the long drive down the East Coast was painful, it would be a serious understatement. There is nothing fun about an overnight road trip with two toddlers who have a strong aversion to being strapped down for three minutes, let alone thirteen hours. We had the expected obnoxious amount of whining and complaining, and too many potty breaks in creepy rest stops. But Disney!!! It would be over soon, and then we could have the time of my . . . I mean, *our* lives.

We pulled in to Orlando, Florida, around 6 a.m., and our major surprise plan unravelled before our eyes. In all of our research, reserving, and ridiculously minute detailing, we kinda forgot that Orlando is a ginormous tourist trap. We saw *giant* fucking Disney billboards *everywhere*. Even for an oblivious little kid, there was no way *not* to see those things.

"Mommy, are we going to Disney?" Holden asked from the backseat.

Shit. Shit shit *shit*!

"No, honey. It's just a billboard advertising for it."

"But why are there so many? Our surprise trip is Disney, isn't it?"

It was then I found myself faced with a dilemma. Do I just come clean, or try to salvage the surprise? Do I *lie* to the kids?? But, lying is *wrong*! I didn't like the idea of being dishonest about something meant to be such a positive moment. But really, this lie was for their own good! I was doing it for the children. Thirteen hours in a car, y'all; I just couldn't give up now.

That's right, I lied my fucking ass off. And judging by the calm and subdued responses from the children, I'd done a damn fine job of it. After I silently congratulated myself for a lie well told, Thomas informed me that we'd be pulling into the resort any minute. This was it; the moment we'd been waiting for! The surprise of a lifetime, the big reveal, our cheesy sentimental family moment. I reached into the bag that sat at my feet and yanked out my handheld video camera, flipped it on, and pivoted around in my seat so that I was facing the boys. This would be a moment to play back when they were teenagers and telling me and anyone who will listen what a horrid biatch I am, and how we never do anything they want to do. In yo' *face*, suckas!

At this point in our long journey, I was giddy, bouncing up and down like a hooker on Ten-Dollar Tuesday. Months of planning and a thirteen-hour drive in the making, and *finally* it was time for the big reveal.

"Guess what, boys?" I asked eagerly, a giant grin across my face.

Both kids looked tired, uncomfortable, and their asses were probably even more numb than mine. They looked over at me and responded flatly: "What?"

"I have something to tell you!"

This was it! Get ready for the peepee parade!

"Our surprise vacation is . . . Disney! We're at Disney World right now!"

As I said this, we pulled through the gate to the resort, just as I'd planned. The whole place was pirate-themed. (Their favorite, duh. Master planner here, remember?) I watched their faces, hoping the giant pirate ship we're driving by will help my words absorb through their thick toddler skulls. But the vague confusion on their faces soon turned into just . . . blah. Nothingness.

"Aren't you excited!? Disney!" I was bouncing again.

Mother of the Year award in 3 . . . 2 . . .

"Yaaaaay . . ."

It was the most forced, weak, and unsurprised "yay" ever.

"Come *on*, guys! Disney! Friggin' *Disney World*! We're here! For a *whole week*!" I was still bouncing, camera still rolling. Someone should have just given me the damn ten dollars so I would stop making an ass of myself.

"Cool."

I deflate and flip off the camera. This was some bullshit! Where was my million-dollar moment??

Yeah, yeah, maybe they were tired, or hungry, or delirious. Maybe I should cut them some slack. Whatever. But I still think they could have faked a mild pant-wetting for their dear old mom.

Despite my epic failure, when all was said and done, we had an absolutely *amazing* vacation that year. Even years later, I still look back fondly on that vacation. I didn't know that when I had kids, it would open up another world to me. One I'd been to before, but wasn't allowed to return to until I spawned my very own womb leech. When you have a kid, you also get to *be* a kid again. You get to do all the things you loved, and all the things you *thought* you'd love but never got the chance to do. Kids can't exactly chaperone themselves, and usually they want you to participate alongside them in the silly, immature, or height restricted things they do, so you can't say no. It's a free pass to immaturity and silliness, and *hell yes* I take advantage of that whenever I can. Whether it's a trip to Disney World, an inflatable bouncy castle, or new toys on Christmas morning—it's all for you! I mean . . . for the kids. A good friend once told me that you might not have a choice when it comes to growing old and saggy, but growing *up* is totally optional. I wish I'd known that from the very beginning—not just of life, but of parenthood. If someone had told me all of this shit from the start, I'd probably have enjoyed my early days as a mom *so* much more.

There's that hindsight crap again. Ugh.

CHAPTER 7

CARTOONS ARE MY CRACK, AND DORA IS MY DEALER

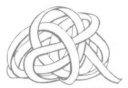

ON VACATION, YOU DON'T HAVE to lift a damn finger. In "real life" there's dishes and dinner and vacuuming. Real life sucks, y'all. And it's hard to get back into the swing of things (a.k.a. domestic slavery) after a vacation. Proof I was getting old? Our fun family vacation exhausted me. Clearly, I needed a vacation after my vacation just to feel relaxed.

Even though I hate to let the kids zone out in front of the TV, when we got back from Disney, I needed some peace and quiet to muster up the strength to do the five tons of laundry stinking up our suitcases. Yet a week without TV can make you forget how *obnoxious* the drivel kids watch these days is. I couldn't sit through more than five minutes of crap-toons before I wanted to jab an icepick into my eye.

When Holden was finally old enough not to sit with a slack jaw and drool pouring out of the corner of his mouth, I began allowing him to watch TV for more than just a few minutes here and there. Quickly, one thing became very clear: Saturday morning cartoons are *not* what they used to be. It was the first time I could say "This just isn't like it used to be" in total seriousness. Let me tell you something: if my kids woke me up on my precious Saturday morning for the junk that comes on TV now, there would be hell to pay. Many species on this planet eat their young, and taking away the small amount of precious sleep I actually get would make me become one of them. I don't know a single parent who doesn't hope that one day, one of these whiny cartoon characters will wander off (because most of them have zero supervision. What the hell?), get bitten by a poisonous snake, and die a slow and painful death. Looking at you, Dora.

I began to take great pleasure in snarking at the television when I was forced to sit through the craptacular nonsense that came on. It was (and still is) my fun little daily ritual and a source of constant amusement. (We all know those moments are few and far between.) Some people yell at sports games, I yell at kids' shows. Don't judge. Here's what a typical Dora-viewing session sounds like at my house:

Stop staring at me; I already answered your stupid ass question!
It's right behind you, moron!
Seriously? Not even you can be that dumb.
Oh come the hell on; as if the parents wouldn't catch on to magical toys in their backyard!?

To think, there are actually times when I find myself wondering where my kids get their back-sassing skills from.

My deep-seated hatred for nearly everything my kids insist on watching has built up over years of unwilling exposure. I hate the nasally voices, the whining, the long awkward pauses, and *all* the lines my corrupt adult brain takes the wrong way. (There are a lot.) The hatred got so intense that I went so far as to ban certain shows from ever appearing on my television for even a split second because they make me grind my teeth so much. But then . . . unpacking needs to be done, or I need to cook and can't get one of the kids out of my anus long enough to get a pot of water boiling, or *I just need to pee, damnit*!

Emergency mind-melting is a necessary evil, even though I swore to the stars in the sky that I would *never* resort to such measures. I felt like a piece of poop for letting my kids reduce their IQs with crap-o-vision, but my house wasn't going to clean itself, and I was too damn tired to be creative. The Supermoms of the world would probably laugh at my failure.

Luckily, my extreme distaste for most things animated was never a secret to the children. They quickly learned not to even *ask* for certain shows or they would incur my ranting wrath. "Oh no, Mommy *hates* that show!" they'd squeal while scrolling the TV guide. But just when you think you have the little vag-nuggets trained to only enjoy what you can tolerate and to not even question it anymore, something very unsettling occurs. Maybe you're sitting on the couch, or standing in the doorway of your living room or bedroom. At that moment, you're completely unaware of your own actions and surroundings because you have been entranced by the glow of the TV. There you are, deeply enthralled by something your wee one watches, a show you have been known to bash relentlessly. The intoxicating pull it has over your brain breaks momentarily; just enough time for you to look around the room and realize that you are alone. *Completely alone*—no children in sight, and they probably haven't been for a solid thirty minutes. In fact, those little a-holes aren't even home.

I have fallen so far down this rabbit hole that one show, which for my itty-bitty ego's sake will not be mentioned by name and which used to be at the very top of my "fuck this shit!" list, slowly started to grow on me. Like a barnacle. Or a giant freaky bunion. I couldn't get away from it. I found myself scrolling through the TV guide to find it, and I would actually get excited if it was on. I didn't want either nugget to find out, or they'd use it against me; kids are terrorists like that. So when I saw this show on the guide,

I would ask the kids if they wanted to watch it, y'know, to make it less weird to flip the TV to that channel. When I'd get the "Ugh, *no*, Mommy!" response, I'd say "Too bad! There's nothing else on!" and I'd put that shit on anyway.

But in reality, other things *were* on. I just had a sickness, and I couldn't control myself. This was not the bottom; not even close. To be honest, it wasn't even the beginning. I was already sinking to even deeper levels of shame. In my darkest hours, when this particular kiddie show would air a new episode during a time that TV watching simply wasn't possible for a small child (like bath time or story time before bed), I would DVR it. Before you start with the "Awwww! What a sweet thing to do!" I have to tell you. . . . I didn't record it for the kids. I recorded it for me. I would wait until the spawn were asleep to watch it. *On purpose. And* I cried.

Look, it was the series finale, and it was sad, damnit! And to be fair, I *did* also watch it with the kids the next day . . . and, of course, I cried. Again.

You'll know you've hit rock bottom when your kids have been in bed for hours, and you're still watching Disney Junior at ten-thirty on a Friday night. Welcome to parenthood. We're all losers here.

CHAPTER 8

WASHABLE, MY ASS!

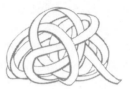

THERE'S ONE GOOD THING ABOUT having two kids with birthdays falling in the same month: it reduces the number of parties I have to throw and times I have to shop for toys. You want time to stand still? Try going to a baby birthday. Sometimes I think we parents only throw these parties to prove to ourselves that there are children out there worse than our own. Shopping for toys is only the *beginning* of the hell that birthdays are, especially with a kid in tow. Taking one into a toy store (or a toy aisle) is just asking for trouble, especially when they know their birthday or Christmas is coming up (and to them, that is *always*). Are you trying to punish yourself? Do you have a death wish? Do you want your child to see every new fifty-dollar gadget that they absolutely *must* have and, if you dare to give in to their demands, will only play with once and never touch again? I'm weak; I've been there. Shit, I'm *still* there. My advice? Avoid! Run away! That's much easier said than done, I know.

After all the time I've spent being taken hostage wandering through aisles of toys, I have come to the conclusion that toys today are insane. That fifty-dollar "I'll only play with this once" gadget? Oh, hell no. Maybe I'm just getting old and I'm used to the rotary toy phone on wheels with the freaky ass face and eyes that follow you and haunt your dreams. You know the one! You'd drag it behind you with the string attached to the front, just begging to be whipped around the house like a weapon. That thing's a classic. And terrifying. Now, when I see it replaced by a toy touchscreen phone with all the bells and whistles, I have to do a double take. It just doesn't seem . . . right. Where's the fear factor??

My kids gravitate toward that crap like bugs to a zapper. They have no idea what half of the junk on the shelves does, but they HAVETOHAVEITRIGHTNOWOMFG-PLEASEMOMMYPLEAAAASE! That's when my inner granny pops out and I actually have to physically restrain myself from saying "Well back in *my* day . . .," but really, things *have* changed. Toy makers have to keep up with the times, I get it. What the hell would a kid do with a flip phone today other than use it as a projectile? Try to explain how a rotary phone works and their heads might explode.

"What the hell is this obsolete crap, Mommy? Now let me throw it at your *face*!"

Little ones *always* want to play with what Mommy or Daddy has; *exactly* what Mommy or Daddy has. It's damn near impossible to satisfy them with a substitution. Toy makers know this and capitalize on it. After far too many sweaty and panicked "where the hell are my keys??" moments caused me to run late to appointments, I gave in. I thought I'd found the equivalent of Willy Wonka's golden ticket by buying Parker, the key-thieving perp, his very own set of keys for Christmas one year.

I'm a genius! Master of parenting! They look and sound just like the real deal! He will never touch my keys again!

As smart, knowledgeable, intuitive, and experienced as we parents are, I swear, sometimes we *never* learn.

Just as I was finishing a round of self-back-patting, the shit hit the fan. Of *course* fake keys weren't going to be acceptable to my tiny dictator. Those damn babies; they might seem like oblivious drooling blobs—*adorable*, but oblivious—but when it comes to attempting to give them decoy toys, somehow they KNOW. Even with similar size, shape, and material—they know! Then, every single time you dare attempt the bait and switch, that tiny drooling face gives you *the look,* touchdown-spikes that shit on the ground, and lets out a wail straight from the depths of hell.

How *dare* you try to fool me, giant stupid human!

Small children may not be able to sense when they're unloading a steaming load of shit into their pants, but they sure as *shit* know that cellphone/set of keys/chunk of your sanity you gave them is a fake. I haven't yet decided if that makes them geniuses, or diabolical masterminds. I fear the latter is more likely, especially when you consider the fact that no matter how well you think you have hidden the real thing, they still manage to get their booger-crusted little hands on it. When it comes to your cellphone, they can *use* it better than you, too. How's that for a kick to the uterus?

The weakness I sometimes feel in the toy aisles came bubbling back to the surface at home. It didn't take long for me to give up being the sole user of my beloved phone, and on always knowing where my keys were at all times— particularly on bad days when nothing else makes those little brats happy (what? I'm not above bribery)—but I didn't quite realize just how far their kleptomania went. Not until I was searching desperately for a tube of ChapStick—which as a female I have a ridiculous cornucopia of—cursing the world under my breath, and I couldn't find a single solitary tube to save my frickin' life. They had vanished! Where the hell could they have gone?

At first I didn't even consider the boys. They'd never taken a lot of interest in my makeup, ChapStick, or really anything overtly "girly" (other than boobs), so why my ChapStick? Why now? I thought that might go down as one of the few mysteries left in the world until one day, while cleaning up the path of destruction left by the boys (because God forbid they clean up after themselves) something caught my eye. No, it wasn't shiny; I'm not a fucking pack rat. I think it was fate that led my eyes to this spot in particular. There, nestled in a pile of arch-slaughtering Legos, was one of my many missing tubes of ChapStick. Before I could rejoice, I pulled the cap off in order to bask in ChapSticky goodness (read: moisturize my poor dry lips) and found what appeared to be primitive teeth markings covering what was left, and giant chunks missing of the rest, rendering my beloved ChapStick completely and utterly useless. Of course, by "primitive," I mean chicklet-sized children's teeth.

Thinking they could outsmart me and hide the truth of what they'd done by burying it in an impenetrable pile of Legos? I think not!

From that moment on, I decided the only thing to do was to have no fewer than fifteen sticks hidden in various places throughout the house. Just in case. How naïve of me to think the pilfering would start with the irresistible jingling of my keys and end with my ChapStick. That was only the beginning of their spree. Maybe it was the rush they experienced from their first ever heist, but soon enough, both kids had turned into full-on thieving hooligans. Nothing was safe! Nothing was sacred! The change in my purse, hair ties, my Freedom nail polish, the TV remote—though my suspicion with the remote is to trap the TV on crap-ass cartoons since changing the channel manually on this new-fangled shit is damn near impossible. Sinister!

Maybe I figured out the mystery of the missing ChapStick, but I will never know how these kids manage to take my stuff right out from under my nose and make it vanish into thin air, never to be seen again. I've even offered ransoms to no avail! Where does it all go? It's a pretty solid assumption to make that when you move out of a house, all that stuff that seemingly poofed into thin air will just as magically appear again and make you feel like an idiot for failing to find it in such an obvious place, like behind the couch or under the bed. Or not. That would just make too much sense. Nine times out of ten, when kids klepto your crap, it is gone *forever*.

Are they in cahoots with the dryer elves? Have they conspired with the Tooth Fairy because she's moved beyond body-part trafficking and we adults are her next victims? Did they *swallow* all of it? Inquiring minds want to know! Inquiring minds do *not*, however, want to sift through poop to find out.

In our house, we have a strict "no markers without supervision" rule after an unfortunate incident with a blue "washable" marker on an eggshell wall (because obviously our landlord hates us and loves walls that no stain can ever be removed from—some men just want to watch the world burn). Kids being kids (read: underhanded and devious), they managed to find a loophole. They *always* find a loophole. I do have to give them credit where credit is due—they got me good. This was one moment that from experience (instead of advice—as stabby as receiving parenting advice makes you) can lead to ugly results.

No, I did *not* tell them in my rage (after Mr. Clean's "magic" couldn't erase their wall art) not to play with pens. I only thought to ban them from the usage of markers since that had been their weapon of choice thus far in life. It was technically my own stupid fault when every single pen in the house disappeared, just like my poor ChapSticks, keys, nail polishes, and sanity. This becomes a real problem when you receive a phone call about an emergency situation where you have to write down important information as it's being relayed to you, which I found out the morning of my father's heart attack. Hospital, wing, room number, phone numbers—all coming at me in a pace so rapid it was hard to keep up. I spun in circles in my kitchen, hands flailing wildly in the air, grasping for a pen that was *not* where I left it. Or the other one. Or the *other* one.

I had to find something, and FAST. What did I have an abundance of? What was strewn all over the kitchen table and counters and ground into the linoleum floor?

Crayons.

After hesitating whether I was really going to write down information that important with colorful wax sticks intended for use on pictures of puppies and kittens, I grabbed one of those fuckers and scribbled down everything I needed to know on a piece of paper . . . which, of course, was completely covered in toddler doodles. What other choice did I have? I was well aware of the puzzled looks from my family as I walked into the hospital with a crumpled piece of paper covered in purple crayon gibberish. Did I care? Maybe a little bit, but that crayon served its purpose—which is *not* being ground into flooring, contrary to what my kids think. I'd say that was the first and last time I'd ever have to go to such desperate measures, but that would be a flat-out lie.

My dad is a trooper. He was out of the hospital in just a few days, and against *my* better judgment (because I control him, didn't he know that?), off to a vacation in Mexico just a few short weeks later. He'd probably *hate* to know how much I worry about him; he doesn't do the whole "man cold" whiny-baby thing many of you men do (Don't shake your head! You know it's true!), so when it came to having to take it easy, well . . . he sucked. After unexpectedly losing my mom right after high school, it was hard *not* to be paranoid. My step-mother takes good care of him, but whenever he comes to visit, the mom-ish me I'd been fighting so hard couldn't help but come out. It was frightening and empowering all at the same time. It came naturally to watch over what he was eating, how much he was eating, and when I saw him exerting himself by picking up Holden's giant bubble-butt, I clenched my teeth and told him to be careful. *Gah, Dad! Just sit down and relax, would ya?* He always looked at me and would say, "You know who you sound like, right?" I pretended not to know, but I knew, and I would scowl—which he would then also say reminded him of my mother. Thanks a lot, Dad. I hope the kids klepto *your* ChapStick! Okay, no I don't. Take it easy!

Sometimes I fondly look back on the days where the only thing within reach when there wasn't a pen in sight was eyeliner or lipstick. Now I can't leave that shit out or it will get stolen, too! Lipstick makes awesome war paint, didn't you know that? Word of advice: buy the cheap shit, or the urge to sell your kids on Craigslist after smearing a thirty-dollar tube of the designer kind all over themselves and the dog may be too overwhelming to resist.

CHAPTER 9

HOW MY VAGINA BIRTHED A NUDIST COLONY

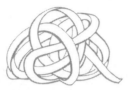

IS IT WEIRD TO WORRY about what my kids are going to remember from their childhood once they get older? Brains hang on to the most random ridiculous nonsense, and the important, yet less "exciting" things get forgotten. Instead of family vacations, will Holden remember the time he had to wear a maxi pad because he had some weird intestinal virus that resulted in sporadic anal leakage? Will Parker forget the time he got down on one knee and proposed to Cinderella, yet remember the day he over-trusted a fart and I had to hose him off in the back yard . . . and it just so happened to be the first day of school during recess, so one hundred little kids just stood there staring at the poop-spraying scene in horror? I'm sure there are more important things to concern myself with, but when I think about what *I* remember, well . . . it's natural to be worried.

If there's one thing I'm never sure of, it's how much recollection of my childhood I am *supposed* to have. You might call that deteriorating mommy-brain (a.k.a. permanent, incurable preggo-brain which consists of forgetfulness, brain farts, and blatant stupidity), but even before I traded in my last functioning brain cells for kids, what I can recall has been left to what I've been told by other family members at gatherings when they were trying to embarrass the shit out of me with a sprinkle of fuzzy "did that really happen?"s and a heaping tablespoon of vivid *might-be* memories. Those are always the ones you wish had been bleached from your brain during your partying years so you could go into parenthood truly thinking there was nothing that would ever eventually bite you in the ass. Unfortunately, it never seems to work out that way . . . at least, not for me.

I remember hating my brother for years because he would constantly hold me down and fart directly in my face—right up the nostrils. I think that's the sole reason I hate hard-boiled eggs to this day. He also got a wild hair up his ass one day and broke my nose; that was pretty uncool. Those are two things I know for *sure* happened. Some things, you just can't un-smell. On the more fuzzy side, from what I've been told, there was a jumper with a smiling blue whale on the front that my mom tried to force me to wear, but I hated it with such a fiery passion that I would scream, cry, and go into banshee mode whenever it came within five feet of me. I may not remember that as vividly as butt-juice up the nose, but at least there's a picture to prove *that* story is true.

The one thing that sticks out in my mind the most are the frightening mental videos that occasionally play back in my head of my mother walking around butt-ass naked in front of me *every single day of my young life*. Every single day! There are no stories being told, no pictures to show as proof, just the knowledge that this *did* happen, and I always wondered *why*? Why would my mother, my own flesh and blood, subject me to such horrors? What could I have possibly done to deserve this retina-burning punishment?

Christ on a bicycle, woman! Why do you hate me so?!?!?

And I remember, just as clearly as her prancing around in the buff, just how much she didn't give a solitary fuck when I expressed my extreme disgust with such an act.

Growing up, I was nothing like my outrageously outgoing, loud-mouthed mother. For the first sixteen years of my life, I was quiet and ridiculously shy, especially when it came to strangers. This shyness spilled over into every aspect of my life. Phone calls? *Hell* no. Public speaking? Avoided like the plague. Peeing in a multi-stall bathroom? Just wasn't gonna happen. Nope! *No one* was to know what the sound of my stream hitting the water sounded like. Not a bit of me would be surprised if everyone in my life thought I constantly had the runs because of how long it would take me to get in and out of a bathroom. It got to the point where my pee-fright became so intense (and stupid) that I would have to run the sink if I knew anyone was within a close enough proximity to hear me go. Even as the shyness faded, I never thought there would be anything that would cure my bathroom bashfulness.

The thought of having to give birth, naked from the waist down, with a room full of people staring up at my stretched-out bits gave me nightmares during pregnancy. Friends and family kept assuring me that I wouldn't care once labor began, but how do you *not* care that a group of strangers, plus the man who *did this to you*, will be seeing you push out a baby . . . and . . . other . . . *stuff*? I don't understand how or why, but they weren't wrong. It all changed the day I gave birth. I was sweaty and disgusting and felt like my private parts had just waged hand-to-hand combat with Chuck Norris. You know, if my vagina had hands. I was so delirious with pain and exhaustion, anything was possible.

To extract Holden's gigantic cranium from my baby chute (which apparently had not been properly greased) I had to be snipped not once, but twice. Imagine a woman's horror upon learning that not only had she stretched out her stomach to epic proportions to make room for this child—but now, quite literally, she was going to have to be cut in half just to get him out. Well, there goes the fun park, I thought. Board that bitch up and mark it as condemned!

In no way shape or form did I want to bear witness to the damage, but after having a nurse manually instruct me on the proper method of flushing my swollen vajay, there was simply no shame left to be found. None. Zilch. Nada. It was then that I sunk to my lowest point. I found myself crying in the hospital room shower because I couldn't bend down to rinse the . . . *birth* . . . off me. I called for the husband unit. Perhaps Thomas felt guilty for being the reason I was in this predicament, because he didn't even object—not even a little.

I found myself weeping with my husband cleaning my gigantic lady-bits and attempting to shave my legs for me. You can imagine how successful that was. I was just glad he didn't catch anything important and chop it off!

That moment may have been the beginning of the chipping away of my parental-denial shell. It may have been small—microscopic even—but once the crack begins, there's no stopping it.

What started as a temporary time-saving method of bathing with baby Holden, one I *swore* I would quit when he got old enough to even attempt to say the word *vagina* (*boobs* is unavoidable), became a five-year stint of communal showering. Look, when you've got one, two, or however many spawn roaming the hallways of your home at any given hour of the day or night, a shower is a *luxury*. I don't like it either, but there's nothing I can do! If I can knock out bathing myself and them at the same time, saving precious minutes *and* money—hell yeah, I'm gonna do it! (Ugh, I sound like a mom.)

In the beginning, I still lived with the notion that other than showers, the bathroom was my sanctuary. I could go there to be alone, collect my thoughts, to pull a "man move" and read on the pot, to just be alone for *once*!

Mobility shattered that dream. Gotta go pee? Suddenly someone is hungry, or stubbed their toe and is on the brink of death, or broke a toy, or kicked something under the couch. Ha! They can wait! I'll close the door! Outsmarted them again! Yeah, no. The door only acts as an amplifier, and then little fingers begin to poke in from under the door and, as if that's not enough to ruin a BM, on turns the whine:

"But mommy! I *neeeeeeeeeeeeeeeeeed* you!"

Getting out a full, satisfying poop was soon a figment of my imagination; something I thought I remembered being real, but like my childhood memories, may have been nothing but lore. Myth. Urban legend. The elusive poop is like the lost city of Atlantis—everyone knows someone who knows someone who knows of its location, but has never witnessed it with their own eyes. The Lost City of Gold to a parent is pushing out a full, uninterrupted turd.

During one boring day in my household, where there may have been whining and a smidge of mayhem, but nothing out of the ordinary, a quiet resolve washed over me. Upon a routine trip to the bathroom to take a typical crappy dump (pun intended), I mindlessly did something different: I left the door open. That's right; letting it rip for the entire house to hear, unlike my pee-fright-filled youth, and just like the butt-naked mom shimmying around in my memories, not a single solitary fuck did I give.

Okay, kids, you want my attention so badly? The bathroom mysteriously morphed into a conference room unbeknownst to me? Fine. I gave up my very last "private" moment, and while using the bathroom will never be the same, I gotta tell ya, you grow quite used to having full conversations while firmly planted on the toilet. The fact that we've rarely had company turned out to be a blessing in disguise, 'cause you better believe that I've grown so used to shootin' the shit while shootin' the shit that I have been known to forget to close the bathroom door while our poor friends and family actually *are* here.

No! I absolutely refuse to believe that motherhood turned me into a full on "Ah, nothing matters anymore! Who cares! I'm a *mom* now!" nudist, lettin' the mom-pooch hang out weirdo, but if you think I'm going to shield my naked vagina from the eyes of two kids who came *out* of it? Well, looks like my mom had the right idea jammin' out with her clam out. Damnit.

She wasn't trying to torture me by walking around in the buff all the time; the simple fact of the matter is that I wouldn't leave her the fuck alone and the woman had to *adapt*!

Sorry, kids. My clam's gonna be jammin' all day every day. My clam is a damn rock star.

CHAPTER 10

OPK (OTHER PEOPLE'S KIDS), AND WHY THEY ARE LIKE FARTS

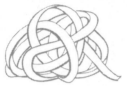

ONE EVENING OUT OF THE blue, my brother sent me a text message and asked if I'd be willing to watch his son for a few hours every week day. According to him, his current childcare provider refused to charge for any less than an eight-hour day, five days a week. He and his baby mama simply didn't need that much care, nor did they want to pay the extra for hours they wouldn't be using, and thought I would be perfect for the job instead. How nice of them to think of me!

I responded by telling him I would need to think about it, but a few seconds later, my phone pinged with another text from my wonderful sibling stating that he'd already told the baby mama I'd said yes, and since they were on rocky terms, he couldn't exactly go back on his word now. Have I mentioned yet how much I *love* my big brother? If you dig deep, I suppose at the end of the day I could have put up a fight about it, but in thinking logically (which I do not enjoy doing), I knew that the extra cash would come in handy, and really—how hard could it be?

My brother's kid, who we'll just call P, is a mere six months younger than Holden. Though the boys didn't spend a *ton* of time together, when they did see one another, they got along famously. To me, P seemed like a pretty good kid . . . as far as kids go, anyway. There wasn't much time to even think about it or prepare myself, because bright and early two days later, little P showed up on my front porch; sippy cup full of juice in one hand, Nutri-Grain bar in the other . . . which promptly reduced to crumbs and exploded all over my living room floor. Complete and utter destruction. Shit.

That was the beginning of three months of pure, nightmarish torture. In part, it had to do with the fact that when you put more than two boys together in one house, they go completely fucking crazy, and the other part was that everything P did drove *me* completely fucking crazy. Don't get me wrong, the kid is my blood and I love the hell out of him, but I'm pretty sure he made my uterus eject from my body and go sprinting into oncoming traffic just to make sure I could never reproduce again on the off-chance that I might have a child similar to him.

How he talked, refused to eat anything other than peanut butter sandwiches . . . the wailing that rivaled an operatic glass-breaking singer . . . emotional outbursts over the tiniest punishments . . . It was maddening, to put it mildly. During that time, I noticed the appearance of my very first gray hairs. Then I got the call from my brother that he was going to be even more frugal and watch P himself during the days and therefore would no longer require my services. Well, let's just say that the only time I've ever been more relieved is after a night of drunken sex, a late period, and a negative pee stick. Hallelujah!

Here's the thing: the kid wasn't actually that bad. P was honestly pretty decent when it comes to kids his age. He just wasn't *mine*. It doesn't take long to figure out that *all* children are obnoxious little creatures who think they are so important that they can wet themselves and someone else will always clean it up. Rude. Every single one of them is a miniature tyrant, hell-bent on world (or maybe just home) domination, and they are *definitely* all attention whores.

It's no secret that for most of my life, the thought of having kids made my vagina recoil in fear; I was just never a child-lover. Didn't want 'em, desire 'em, want to wash the asses of 'em. Don't even *ask* me when I'm having one of my own because that nonsense is *not* happening for *so* many more reasons than just the ones listed above. I wasn't about to be a servant to someone who can't even manage to hold a spoon horizontally, let alone know when they were going to projectile vomit all over the nearest face. Although I absolutely loved money growing up, you still couldn't even convince me to babysit. I could not stand those little brats, and all parents knew it by the disgusted/annoyed/horrified look on my face whenever one of their creatures was in my presence. To be fair, they didn't seem to like me much, either. It was a mutual dislike, and I was okay with that. Well, as long as I didn't have to hear them. Or smell them. Just keep them away!

"Oh, it's so much different when they're your own!" people even as far back as my mother would say—and I would respond by snorting in their faces. Yeah, right! Whining is whining no matter who it's coming out of, or who made the creature doing the whining. All of it is annoying! I don't care if the one making that wretched noise just so happened to drop out of me!

Oh ye of little faith.

Cut to years later, after I'd experienced the pain of labor firsthand and dealt with a child who thought the rising of the moon meant he had to howl at it. And the sun. And the clouds. Okay, what I'm saying here is he screamed *All. The. Time.* He wasn't a werewolf; he was a baby with reflux. Pretty much the same thing if you ask me. I'm pretty sure reflux babies magically created an extra hour in the day just so they could scream during it. It was every kind of awful you can imagine. I was tired and irritated and didn't even have time to eat most days because I was so busy trying to stop his incessant cries, but he was *my* baby; my sweet, fat-roll-covered baby. My *perfect* creation. I spent a number of miserable hours writhing around in a hospital bed with people seeing every part of me in the most unflattering light just to explode him out of my poor unsuspecting lady bits. My can-do-no-wrong baby. Damnit. Those evil parents were right! His whining and crying wasn't nearly as annoying as the whining and crying from other kids simply because he was mine and they were not. And that is saying something, since he *never* shut up!

After months of those long nights rocking my Werebaby to sleep, it was my turn be the one at the store with the screeching child. I found myself looking around at the childless buttholes who were cringing like I once cringed and realized just how wrong I had it, and how much of a judgmental asshole I had been. From that point on, if I heard another kid screeching and howling? I thanked the stars in the sky it wasn't mine and would give a sympathetic "I have *sooo* been there and feel your pain" look to the frazzled parent trying to subdue the mini-beast. Solidarity, sister! Or brother . . . whichever. You get the point. It's pretty amazing what one look of sympathy can do for the parent feeling like the worst fucking parent in the world.

And then, right in the middle of my non-judgy understanding solidarity came the moment we all have because we are nothing more than mere humans. Once again, we hear the oh-so-familiar sound of a scream from a baby, or a small child . . . or possibly a velociraptor . . . ringing through the aisles. Some kid, somewhere, is having a full-on shit-fit meltdown, and instead of throwing my fist up and shouting "Yaya!" I realized exactly what those parents meant when they said "it's different when it's your own."

Here, all this time, I thought the point was that I would be able to tolerate my own even at their worst moments because I grew their nasty little asses, and love extends far beyond the pain tolerance and patience thresholds. Nope. The truth is really that other people's kids are not mine, and that's where the line is drawn. I have built up a tolerance to the chicanery and downright jerky behavior that has been bestowed upon me every day since plopping out a kid. I am *not*, however, used to someone *else's* kid's chicanery and jerkiness. If you catch me at an off (read: irritable) time? Holy shit. *That* kid is annoying as hell! I'm so glad *my* kids aren't that annoying! Is it possible to shove that thing back up into your hooha? Because you really should. It would at least muffle the noise coming out of them!

The thing is . . . they are. My kids *are* that annoying! Just not to me. It's even quite possible that they are even *more* annoying than the little shit bellowing down the frozen foods aisle that has been dancing a jig on my very last nerve—but I'm used to it. *Frighteningly* used to it. Being *that* used to the absurd amount of bratty behavior that goes on in our homes every day is like being used to someone repeatedly sawing off your leg with no anesthesia. And then beating you with it. Repeatedly. Maybe we should praise ourselves daily for being so strong in the face of pure evil.

It was a scary point in my life when I finally processed just how deluded I had become when it came to how obnoxious my kids really are. It might just be the ultimate level of asshole filling the confines of my home each and every day, and I'd never even realized it because I'd convinced myself that every kid on this planet is more annoying than mine. It's not my fault! Those heathens didn't occupy my insides. That's what forced me to love my own no matter what. I don't have a choice! Even through the most obnoxious of whines, they can't drive me to *total* insanity like the product of someone else's genitals can.

"It's different when it's your own kid." Ugh. Is it possible to be allergic to parenting advice? There's not much on this planet that I dislike more than being told how I'm supposed to feel, what I'm supposed to do, or whether I'm doing something right when it comes to my own children. Yes, many people just think they're helping, but unless I specifically *ask*, I don't wanna hear it! It made me feel so disconnected from other parents to always be drowning in unsolicited advice that I never thought fit me or applied to my life and kids. It pained me more than a razor cut in the bikini zone to swallow my pride and admit that *any* advice dispensed to me by other parents was true, but I couldn't refute this one. That irked me even more. There I was, not understanding the mindset of the stereotypical Supermom at all, and then they had to go and say something I agreed with. How dare they! Bastards.

Yes, all of our kids are annoying and we love them anyway, and *always* more than the more annoying, yet less annoying kid next to them. There's a saying I heard a few years ago that still stands the test of time: "Kids are like farts: you can handle your own, but others' are *unbearable!*"

I once dated a guy who would fart these nasty rotten-egg clouds and announce proudly, "Everyone likes their own brand!" It was one of the many reasons I couldn't see a future with him (probably due to anus-cloud fog), but he was right. So were those damn advice-giving know-it-all parents. The only advice I have ever found to be anywhere near as true as that one is never to wear white pants while Aunt Flo is dropkicking down your uterine door.

CHAPTER 11

Tears are contagious. So if you start crying, I will have to spray you in the face with Lysol.

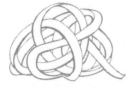

When I was about seven years old, the family dog was diagnosed with cancer and shortly thereafter had to be put down. I know; what a bummer! Who starts a chapter that way? I'm sorry!

My parents came home from the vet and broke the news to my brother and me, who had stayed behind with our grandparents. When I didn't cry, I found my little ass in a giant pot of scalding water. They actually *grounded* me for not crying—*that* made me cry. It's not that I was insensitive or cold; of course I loved that dog. I just wasn't sentimental or sappy. If my brother stole one of my toys to blast apart in the backyard a la Sid from *Toy Story* then *that* would end in tears. Happily ever afters and dying animals? Just didn't do it for me. I guess that's why I never understood growing up what all the hoopla about how terribly sad *Bambi* was. The mother being shot was so insignificant to me that all I could really remember is Thumper. I loved the shit out of Thumper.

My teenage to young adult years weren't much better. I heard friends going on and on about some sappy love-story movie and how it was the most romantic and heartbreaking thing they had ever seen, and that they cried so hard watching it they blew snot bubbles. Yeah, I made

51

that last part up, but really—that's how huge of a deal they were making of it. After hearing about something so many damn times, even from guys who were actually admitting to tearing up themselves, I had to see it for myself. I was expecting greatness. Would my Grinch-y heart grow three sizes that day?

No. The answer is no, it did not. I did not "Get Notebooked," as the kids called it. The only reaction it got out of me was a lot of sighing from utter boredom and groaning at the extreme cheesiness. I could feed an entire elementary school grilled cheese sandwiches with the overflowing cheese-level of that craptacular movie. If it weren't for the eye candy in the form of Ryan Gosling (Hello, nurse!), there's no way I would have made it to the end without throwing things at the screen or digging out my eyes with spoons just so I wouldn't have to watch any more of it.

Was I broken? Why couldn't I cry at sappy movies? Is my heart *really* tiny, cold, and black? I wondered if perhaps I should put STEAL CHRISTMAS on my To-Do list. It truly sucked to be the only one not crying like a baby. Maybe that sounds weird; I just wanted to be included, even if I frequently giggled at all the silly girls with their silly tears. Clearly, I was a man's woman! Or . . . a woman's man? A hard-core kick-ass biatch! I was tough!

Once I went and got myself knocked up, I guess the excess body fat I quickly packed on melted the ice around my heart. Almost immediately, along with extreme irritability and freakish sausage toes, I found myself getting weepy over pretty much everything. Most notably, a cartoon. Not some super-sappy family-oriented miracle on some numbered street crap, or even poor Bambi; it wasn't even anything with any real sentimental value. I was choking up over *Futurama*, a cartoon intended to make toilet humor loving adults laugh. Who cries at that?? Pregnant, waddling, pee-my-pants-when-I-sneeze, hormonal mess me, that's who. I was so sad watching it that I was on the verge of *sobbing*. Talk about completely out of control!

I'd hoped the newfound emotional junk attacking my insides I had experienced so intensely while pregnant was a fluke. A phase. Just a one-time thing, never to happen again—like the time I ate an entire pizza by myself, or the time I stuck a thousand forks in my crush's front yard and nearly got arrested. Just once, it doesn't need to repeat itself! Once I evacuated my uterus, the problem would solve itself, and I could go back to my cold, uncaring self, snort-laughing at the emotional females. Oh! I know! Maybe it was an allergic reaction to dust! That's totally possible! I hadn't dusted in a while because my giant preggo ass wasn't even supposed to get out of bed unless I needed to take a dump.

Much to my chagrin, the "womanly" emotional moments that I had rarely, if ever, experienced before I started growing my very own miniature human only got *worse* once I popped. Just when I thought there was no way for it to get any *more* terrible than having to fan my face with my hands after watching a frickin' diaper commercial with "You Are My Sunshine" playing softly in the background because I was so overcome by these disgusting things called *feelings*, I had another baby. Damnit!

Fireworks at Disney World? Total weepy baby moment. Fireworks! What the heck? *Any* commercial or show where a kid grows up and leaves for college, moves away, or takes a trip to the store while the mom or dad (or both) sadly watches them go? Forget about it! I can't keep myself together. Seeing a semi-terrible actor "tear up" (the ones where you are almost certain they were sprayed in the face with a water bottle right before the director called "action!" because it seems so fake)? My eyes instantly start to burn and water. Do not bring super-sappy over-the-top cheesetacular "chick flicks" to my house; no, not even the one I used to tease people for crying over. Get the fuck outta here with that! I can't handle it! I'm coming apart at the seams!

To be frank, I was downright mortified by this intense hormonal and all-too-stereotypical woman thing I had going on, especially when it happened around Thomas. He's seen two babies get yanked from my nether region while it was stretched beyond anything anyone should ever have to see (and all while I was screaming "Stay above the shoulders!"), but I still don't want the man seeing me transform into a clichéd, crazy, sentimental, weepy woman.

I never wanted to have to say "it's a woman thing, you wouldn't understand" or pull out my lady card as an excuse to why I was acting a certain way (be it good or bad). In my opinion, other than the things that hang off us, men and women really aren't all that different. Stupid fucking hormones ruined that for me! I'm aware that men are capable of and even *do* sometimes cry . . . but most of them won't ever do it around anyone else once they are past the age of ten. I don't know how they manage it. It must have something to do with a lack of vagina-y influence coursing through their systems left behind by a dropped placenta.

Vagina has a *much* different influence on the male species.

We ladies get the privilege of being the gender that carries our young. We get to feel them move, all those kicks and the Tae Kwon Do practices they have up in that bitch. We even get to form a bond with them before they take their first breath, which is all pretty darn awesome, but we got the shit end of the stick when it comes to psychotic emotions. At merely the *thought* of trying to conceive, there should be an alarm that sounds: *Danger! Side effect: Brain will unhinge immediately upon fertilization!*

Estrogen is evil. What I'm saying here is that you dudes out there are the lucky ones.

Maybe estrogen is not the real reason. I'm no doctor or scientist, and all I really do is write whatever crazy idea comes to my head, but I do know that Thomas is never crying and I am *always* crying, and I never want him to catch me crying because then he will think I have gone and lost my damn mind . . . and he will be absolutely right. Damn kids and their damn life-changing effects!

Things haven't gotten any better over time, either. To me, it made sense that the more days, weeks, months, *years* that had passed since the last time I gave birth, the weaker those wacky pregnancy and post-partum feelings would get. My uterus would lose her hold over my brain and go back to only being able to torture me for one week out of every month (which is still a lot if you ask me). Probably just to spite me, instead of fading into the wild blue yonder, they continued to grow. Like a weed. Or genital warts.

I can't even get through an hour of television without my eyes burning or boogers running. All those pregnancy books that I thought I *had* to read only prepared me for my nose getting wider and stretch marks. I had even accepted that my hips were just never going to go back down to their pre-pregnancy size, but I had no idea becoming a parent meant I would be reduced to a puddle of mush over bad dramatic acting—and not because it was bad enough to weep for the future of television and cinema! Add this to the ever-growing list of things to thank my children for.

On the plus side, my stoic husband who shed no tears because he is a "Man's Man," and manly men do not cry at such nonsense that hysterical overdramatic women do, has actually started to crack, just like me. Sympathy hormones? Behind his back, I call him Humpty-Dumpty because once he finally cracks, no one is going to be able to put him back together. Then he'll be a big fat crybaby, and no longer will

I be alone in this ridiculousness. The kids may not have come out of his vagina, but that doesn't mean he can't act like he has one. Phantom vag—just another side effect of parenthood for men.

I have witnessed him get sentimental over things he used to laugh at me for being bothered by. Superman's Man can't watch *Law & Order: SVU* anymore, just like me, and although he would deny it, while watching some of our favorite shows, I have most definitely heard him let out an "awww," or a "that's so sad." I think I even saw him tear up over the same family show that I have to mentally prepare myself to watch because every damn week it makes me bawl. (If you've never watched *Parenthood*, don't say I didn't warn you.) The times that I had to unwillingly bark "I'm a woman!" at him when he quizzically stared over at me because I was rapidly fanning my eyeballs trying to keep the tears in were quickly coming to an end! Hallelujah! I see the fucking light!

One day Humpty Dumpty will fall and girly cry, but for now he values his testicles too much to allow them to be sucked up into his body and transform into ovaries so large there is simply no more room and liquid is forced out of his tear ducts. One day! For now, it's just me who is the loud, embarrassing mess. That's okay, though. If I can wait hours for two kids to get the hell out of my birth canal, I guess I can wait a little longer for Thomas to break.

CHAPTER 12

NO, I AM NOT SMARTER THAN A FIFTH GRADER. NOT EVEN CLOSE.

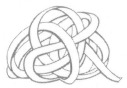

I'VE HAD A STARTLING NUMBER of self-realizations since I stopped only caring about myself and put the most obnoxious, yet ridiculously cute humans in my life first. Oh, and I guess my husband is okay, too, but I was referring to the kids; the *kids* come first. I don't like the term *high maintenance* when it comes to my former years, because what comes to mind is a prissy snob who thinks five minutes can be stretched to an hour and no one should be upset about it, but I was certainly no slouch. I liked to take a shower at least twice a week and I preferred my meals hot, is that such a crime?

With two little mouths open and squawking like obnoxious, hairless baby birds, hot meals are a thing of the past. Turns out, lukewarm isn't so bad. I haven't seared off any taste buds with food fresh off the stove and hotter than molten lava in years. Perspective! I've also realized that my definition of *dirty* may have been a *bit* too strict before kids. More than that, I have zero interest in doing forty-seven loads of laundry every single week—so you're going to have to wear those pants one more time before I'll consider washing them. For me, the most essential thing to figure out when it came to clean or dirty, hot or cold, work smarter or work harder, was *never* to put things to the "smell test." Ever. Trust me on this.

When I was only doing my own laundry, I already knew and was used to most, if not all, of the . . . *aromas* that waft and permeate from my skin. Other people? Look, you don't want to smell other people's aromas. Unless you enjoy the stench of a rotting anus, or the putrid fragrance of week-old shart, do *not* put another human's (no matter how small they are) clothes up to your nose and inhale. Consider this a PSA: if you question its cleanliness, put it *directly* in the washer. Do not pass go. Do not collect two hundred dollars.

These were things I knew; facts not to be argued with. One whiff and you'll learn not to *ever* do that again. Another thing I had become aware of was—even if it pained me to accept it—that even with as much as I'd learned over all of my years on this planet, I would never know enough to not feel like I didn't know a damn thing when it comes to children. Parenthood isn't a video game you can level up in. A game show, however, now *that* I could see!

Some years back, there was this game show that everyone was crazy about where adults would try to answer questions that came straight from elementary school curriculum. It was hosted by a man that many people considered charming and honest when it came to just how intelligent he was: Mr. Jeff Foxworthy. Just to refresh your poor, tired memories (or maybe that's just me), if the adults got the questions right, they'd win money. If they didn't know the answer, there would be an entire panel of ten- to eleven-year-olds to give them what *they* thought the correct one was. About 95 percent of the time, the kids knew a hell of a lot more than the adults. It was funny to watch, but pretty embarrassing to see adults, who are supposed to be smart and the ones *teaching* these children, getting totally smoked by ten-year-olds. The show was called *Are You Smarter Than a 5th Grader* and if you ask any high school or college graduate that question, the obvious response is yes, of course! I'm older, wiser, and have more education under my belt!

Most days I may have felt like I was beating my head against a wall trying to find where I fit in this whole weird "parenting" thing, but you didn't need to put me on a TV show in front of the entire fucking country for me to know whether I'd beat a fifth grader in a battle of wits. The answer is no! Hell to the no! I've been out of school for too long, done too many things that have probably killed half my brain cells. (Uh, hello? Children! What, you thought I meant drugs? Psh!) Meanwhile, kids are busy having knowledge crammed into their spongy brains by trained professionals. Unfair advantage.

No, I am not smarter than a fifth grader, and on most days, I get outsmarted by my own little kids. They aren't even in fifth grade yet. As I write this, one isn't even in school yet! How do ya like them apples? I don't like them at all, personally. There we are, going through ten months of hell and however many long hours of beyond-threshold pain bringing them into this world, and they turn around and make us feel like complete idiots by their fourth years on this planet. Yes, I just wrote fourth. And that's being conservative.

Way to bite the hand (or boob) that feeds you, brats!

Long gone were the days where Holden could be easily outsmarted and outwitted because he was too slow to come back with anything other than "but . . . but . . . but . . ." Memories, oh how I cherish them! By four years old, he was using an array of different tactics to get what he wanted or to get himself out of trouble (which he found his sassy ass in a lot). Many times, I had trouble arguing with him, because damnit, he made too much sense.

On his first attempt, he tries what I like to call "whore logic."

What is "whore logic"? Redefining the parameters of a situation to justify an awful action, or to claim something is true that is patently untrue, usually in order to preserve your image in the face of others; e.g., "I've only slept with four guys . . . if you don't count vacation sex, one night stands, drunk sex I don't remember, or those guys I don't like anymore."

Whores and small children; who knew they had so much in common?

Everything is okay if you can ignore reality and put a spin on it that benefits no one but you. No, I didn't push Parker on purpose! I did it because he was looking at me the wrong way and I was just trying to get him to look at something else, so I was only helping! Never mind the fact that he wasn't actually looking at me, and wanted nothing to do with me, and I shoved him just to be an asshole and you witnessed the whole thing. It's still not my fault. Not completely!

Good ol' fashioned whore logic strikes again. It's just too bad for him that even at my dumbest, most forgetful moments, I never *ever* fall for it.

Once whore logic inevitably fails, he would switch tactics and argue his case like a well-seasoned defense lawyer. Case-in-point: Holden wanted to take his indoor toys to play outside—the things that would likely get ruined if shoved into the dirt and then rubbed across grass. In no uncertain terms, I told him no, that his idea simply wasn't going to happen. Hell to the no, because inside toys stay *inside*. Duh. His response?

"Well, at the end of *Toy Story 3* that girl and that boy play with inside toys outside and that was okay."

Touché, evil little genius. Curse that Walt Disney!

I had absolutely no response because he was totally right . . . and because I was amazed at how well he outsmarted me. He had fucking reference material to back him up! But I still said no. That's animated, not real. Doesn't count, sorry! Actually, I'm not really sorry. When even his outsmarting doesn't work, he pulls out the trump card. He does the one thing he *knows* will either get him exactly what he wants or immediately diffuse whatever situation is about to serve him his own ass on a platter. He used a Jedi Mind Trick. Yes, he used the fucking Force.

On one particular afternoon, Holden was on my damn nerves more so than he is on any other typical day. At one point during that time, I caught him staring at me. Just staring. The boy put on the whole "I'm a kid and many adults find that terrifying, which is why little kids are used in nearly every single scary movie, only solidifying their creepy status once and for all"—a concept used in way too many horror films. I'm sure many fellow parents are aware how irritating and unnerving that can be—right up there with "Mom! Mommy! Mama! Ma! Mommy!" Being that I had already had my fill of his shenanigans that day, I snapped. "Why are you staring at me?" That was when he came back with the ultimate mind-fuck: "Because . . . nobody stares at anybody when they stare." Instantly, I felt a sense of calm wash over me. I couldn't even remember what I was mad about. He beat me. Fair and square. The little shit finally won.

Nope, I definitely don't need a TV show to tell me I'm not all that smart. That all of my years in school were completely pointless because all that's left in my brain are fart jokes, knowing how to take off my bra without taking off my shirt first, and the lyrics to the theme song of Spongebog Fucking Squarepants. My kids have done a mighty fine job of proving that all on their own.

CHAPTER **13**

I HOPE YOU STEP ON A LEGO

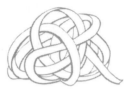

THE SUMMER BEFORE HOLDEN'S FIRST year of school was a rough one. I was slightly (read: completely) freaking out that my baby, who I'd spent every waking moment of the last five years with, would now be gone all day long. He was my best buddy, my partner in crime, and he was soon going to be gone for six hours a day, five days a week. I wasn't ready to let go yet, damnit! And I wasn't sure if Parker and I would even get along without a third party to act as a buffer. Terrible twos, y'all; the struggle is real.

Those last few months were the roughest on Parker, whose head was tragically far too big for his body (hereditary, as I too am a human Pez dispenser) and would constantly throw him off balance. But no matter how many times I told him to put his HANDS OUT to catch himself when he felt he was losing his hold of gravity, he never did.

That entire summer was spent with Parker's lip busted and disgusting. Any time it would heal, his cranium would get the better of him and down he'd go again, smacking his face in the *same* spot on the concrete patio in the back yard—no hands used to break the fall. His face broke his fall. It was gruesome. The poor kid just couldn't win, and as terrible as I felt for him . . . well, he only had himself to blame. Had he just *listened to mommy*, his precious chubby-cheeked face would have remained scab free. One or two times of this whole "not listening" business and I'll still coddle someone. After that, it's your own damn fault! If I've told you specifically, repeatedly, sternly, "Do *not* do that or bad things will happen!" and you choose not to listen after the bajillionth time? Well, my sympathy goes away and is replaced by something else. Actually, it kind of felt like some*one* else.

It seems a million years ago when I look back at my first childbirth experience, and even though I have tried my hardest to block some things out of my memory (Um, hello? Swollen lady parts? I'd rather not have that visual seared into my brain forever), there are some things that just stuck with me. Like caramel in my teeth, or accidentally putting on a maxi pad tape side up. When I was in labor with Holden, I kept wondering why on earth the nurse assigned to me kept rolling her eyes whenever I requested something for the incredible pain I was experiencing. Instead of making it easy and saying yes, she would ask me, on a scale from one to ten what my current level of pain was and I'd reply with an angry "Six!"

Six is pretty fucking bad! Am I right? Especially in the giant uncomfortable area that contained a baby. Comparatively, in my mind, six is on the verge of tears kind of pain. More than stubbing your pinky toe on a table but less than, say, falling out of a tree into a pit of rusty nails. *Give me something for it right now, damnit! Put that needle in me! Just the tip! Just for a minute!!*

I realized once I was in full-blown—baby flying down the hatch at warp speed and *someone* had better be down there to catch it *right now*—labor, shouting "Thirteen!" at this poor woman, and seeing the look of "that's more like it" on her face, that six was *nothing*. Certainly *she* already knew that, having witnessed who the hell knows how many births, but how was *I* to know that a pain level of six was nothing more than child's play? I felt kinda bad about all the horrible things I called her under my breath when I thought she was just trying to torture the whiny overdramatic pregopotamus for her own sadistic pleasure. After that, my entire outlook on pain changed. No longer was there a simple one-to-ten pain scale to consider. It would never be that easy again.

I have had mono with bronchitis, fevers so high that I was completely delirious and seeing talking slugs, broken nearly every finger, and we can't forget the multiple times I was hurt after getting an ass-whooping from an older brother who enjoyed nothing more than expressing his sibling rivalry with a Charlie horse and fart to the face. Not to mention the kidney infections and a spiral fracture of my left leg that was so bad my foot was literally on backwards. All of those things I would have considered a level-ten pain—none of which even came *close* to comparing to childbirth. Mind officially blown.

No longer could I measure pain the same way I had been instructed to my entire life. There was no more one to ten. There was just one—childbirth. No *way* could I say that childbirth was just a measly ten, especially not looking at those stupid pain charts in every doctor's office where their cheaply drawn version of the worst pain you have *ever* felt in your entire fucking life was nothing more than a frowny face with one little tear.

Where was the puffy redness? The snot pouring with a blubbering bottom lip? The "I just ran a mile with a baby in my birth canal" swollen face? The broken blood vessels like you lost a bar fight? The gritting of teeth? The horrified look of "what the hell is *happening* to me?" Where in the holy hell was the string of expletives in a thought bubble over the head? What about the drawing of a wide open screaming mouth that occurs while a baby claws and shreds its way down the birth canal? If I am to believe that

Mr. Frowny Face is supposed to indicate the "worst pain I've ever experienced," there had *better* be a wide open screaming mouth at the very least!

This newfound enlightenment, I would soon learn, really clouded my responses and compassion toward others when they claimed they were in pain (as in the case of Parker and the pavement). Thanks a lot, parenthood. As though my hormones didn't make me enough of a bitch by themselves!

Husband complains of skull-crushing headache? Please. I pushed an almost eight-pound child out of my *vagina*. Twice! Doctor wants to know how much pain I'm in from tweaking my back while helping my kid down a water slide? Well, shit. Yeah, it hurts—but if we're comparing it to birthing a human—it doesn't even come close! I left that appointment with nothing to help my pain. Sonofa biscuit! Kid falls down and is boo-hooing about how their leg is absolutely going to need to be amputated? I sure do love you, and I'll kiss it to make it better . . . but seriously? Doctors had to snip my va-jay-jay *twice* to pull your gigantic skull out of it. Did you ever stop to consider that?? Shut your face-hole, whiner!

I'm honestly surprised my family hasn't divorced me and then filled my spot with a more sympathetic maternal figure by now. I can't help the truth! And I can't help that once you give birth to something larger than even the *worst* post-constipation rock-hard turd, everything else seems like child's play . . . and let's not even *talk* about recovery pain. I most *certainly* can't help that everyone else suddenly sounds like a bunch of bellyaching babies. As if my house needed another one of those.

People will try to tell you that once you have your child in your arms and begin to watch them grow, you will forget all about the pain and absolute horror you experienced bringing them into this world. Those people are filthy fucking liars. I guarantee the *only* reason that particular memory fades is because those little turds melt your brain until it can't remember farther back than three days. No matter how hard you try to block it out, or your beaten up female parts try to force you to forget so you'll get duped into doing it again, you will always remember that deep down, childbirth (and probably the few weeks preceding and following it) is the most awful pain anyone could ever feel. There is truly nothing else that compares. Actually, I take that back. There is only *one* other thing that comes even remotely close to the pain of labor and delivery. It is a sharp, searing, and mind-altering pain. And much like childbirth, it *changes* you.

Out of the blue one day, you will probably find yourself saying "unless you've just birthed a child or stepped on a Lego, don't come crying to me about pain!" Life drastically shifts when you have the intimate knowledge that the only pain even close to shoving a baby out of your hoo-ha is stepping on a tiny plastic block. My living room is a battle zone. I don't dare walk through it without the lights on; I'm not that brave! The sad part is, it's still not even close to squeezing a tiny human out of your vagina at all! There *was* one time my ear got so infected that it *felt* like it was giving birth . . . alas, once it was over, there were no stitches, or enormous pads resembling adult diapers full of ice needed. Labor still wins, with honorable mention going to Barbie shoes. Fuck those things and the pink convertible they rode in on!

CHAPTER 14

Nobody puts baby in a corner . . . unless baby is a drunken mom who never gets out

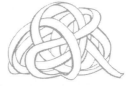

THANKS TO THAT WONDERFUL THING we call the Internet, I received the news via Facebook that my ten-year high school reunion was only a few months away. My first thought was, "Holy *balls*, I'm old!" My second thought was "has it really been ten years already?" If you think your friends having kids on purpose ages you, try realizing that you've been out of high school for a decade. Process that shit! I didn't want to! *Ten* years. Wow.

In ten years I had graduated, lost my mom, moved to California and back, gone on tour of the east coast as a musician, lived with all kinds of skeevy, disgusting, and annoying roommates (and dated even skeevier ones), gotten married, and had not one, but *two* kids. To make it short: life had changed. With all of those changes in just ten years, it's easy to imagine I lost contact with a *lot* of the people I'd gone to school with. It didn't matter that I'd spent years in the same building with my classmates—when you don't keep in touch and aren't forced to see each other every day, after so many years, you don't really know each other at all. Eighteen years old compared to twenty-eight is a world of difference . . . or at least, you *hope* so. You hope that just as you had realized that you were a raging asshole or mega-bitch, others had come to their senses and grown the hell up, too, and any negative feelings were water under the bridge.

It's not like I'm a shining beacon of maturity or anything—but I certainly don't spend my spare time gossiping about someone's skanky butt-cheek baring shorts or heinous hairstyle. Not *all* of my spare time, anyway. I definitely don't spend my time in the school library photocopying dirty notes that an underclassman wrote to my crush and then taping it up in every single hallway and then proceeding to drop a whole stack of them over her head from the upper level. Yes, I really did that. Like I said, MEGA-bitch.

I had since seen the error of my ways and had reformed. I was a stay-at-home mom who had taken up a career in writing now. I was a respectable, contributing member of society! That at least had the *assumption* of maturity to it. Most of my classmates had no idea what I was doing with my life, nor I them. Even though I'd helped to plan the whole event from beginning to end, and had somehow accepted the role of co-host, I was going in blind, and a little scared to be honest. Okay, a LOT scared. But I was also really excited.

Thomas and I had not been out alone together very often since Holden was born. What I mean by "not very often" is twice in *five* years, and both times turned out to be disastrous. The first time, my friend who was sitting (just baby Holden at the time) decided it would be fun to wake him at midnight to play with him—making me paranoid to ever leave him with anyone other than Thomas again . . . and even *that* was a stretch. So what if I'm baby-clingy??

The next was years later during a family trip. My cousin was gracious enough to take pity on our sad and lacking social life situation and sat in the hotel room with the boys while they slept so Thomas and I could go out as a couple. That was cut short by a hideous, rashy allergic reaction I'd broken out in due to the hot Florida sun and my inability to do anything other than fry even with SPF one-friggin'-hundred on. When we got back to the room, we found Holden naked and pretty much every square inch of the room caked in barf. Hooray for food poisoning! That was a *long* night and even *longer* next day, since my ass up and decided it wanted to participate in the fun, as well.

We were cursed. That's the only illogical logical explanation that fits. Any time my poor husband and I got out alone, something *always* went wrong. Maybe we were just meant to be homebodies! Most nights I didn't even mind not getting to go out to dinner, or to a bar, or the movies, but I had busted my *ass* on this reunion. There was no way I was missing it. And no *way* was I going without my husband as a date. It had been too damned long.

When reunion night finally came, after the hour it took to make myself presentable to the general public (read: *hot enough to make former classmates question whether or not I was telling the truth about popping out a handful of kids*), I was thrilled to fling myself out the front door! Free at last! One last check in the mirror (which would probably make the five thousandth) and instead of saying "Good enough, I guess," I actually felt like I looked good, and for the first time in a long time, I felt like me. Not the me *before* kids, and not the apprehensive one after, but a confident woman—a writer and mother—a different me.

After my friend who had so graciously agreed to watch the boys arrived and I gave him a run-down of how our evenings usually go while trying not to panic, we nervously left them and were on our way. I was ready to let loose and have a good ass time like the olden days; only now I didn't have to worry about ending up with some creepy douche at the end of the night since I had a husband on my arm. He may be a douche, but he's *my* douche, and there would be no walk of shame. Winning!

My ten-year high school reunion with a husband by my side and two kids safely at home with a babysitter—how mature and adult-like of us! How completely fucking weird . . . but in a good way for once.

Once we got there, it was the typical reunion setting. There was a table with nametags, a small hotel ballroom, and people who only recognized each other by the sticker proclaiming "Hello! My name is . . ." while squinting at older-looking faces and exchanging awkward pleasantries and short stories about what they filled the years with since high school. The best part, in my opinion, was that the ballroom was right next to the hotel bar. Score! Bring on the adult beverages! Mama doesn't have to drive tonight! I was relieved to find out that I was not the only parent, but soon came to learn that it did leave me with a stigma on my back. Or maybe my forehead. Yeah, probably my forehead. It was giant, neon, and blinking—and totally sucked. Party poopers as far as the eye can see! Why does someone always have to pee in the communal Cheerios?

There I was, busy chatting up old acquaintances while eating a fabulous dinner that I didn't have to cook (cha-ching!), slurping down drinks like I would assume people at reunions were supposed to do, but my excitement to actually be out of the house without my two babies, replaced by a newfound sense of non-bitchy social butterfly persona (also known as "loud") had people whispering. Being an inexperienced heel-wearer, my "fuck-me pumps"—after a few hours of walking back and forth, getting people their raffle tickets, and attempting to host an event that I had *no* damn idea how to host—began to make my feet ache. This led to wobbling, and to me, a strut that may have looked like I needed to take a dump, but to others like I was totally wasty-face, pole-dancing drunk.

"First time out of the house in a while, huh? You must really be letting loose!"

Wait, what? I was puzzled. I was only being myself, well . . . the myself without ankle-biters dangling from my pant legs. What was I supposed to be acting like, exactly?

"You're gonna feel that in the morning! Take it easy, *Mom*!"

Excuse me? Feel what? My feet aching? Well duh! Tired from staying out late because I never go out? No shit, Sherlock! And what does being a mom have to do with anything? Were they implying that since I have kids, it means Mom is all that I am? Oh *hell* no.

As if I wasn't having enough of my own issues learning to really feel like the title of "mom" was a part of who I was, it was thrown in my face as though it was something to be embarrassed about. As if it means I can't do anything other than wiping butts and kissing booboos. I was pissed. This was exactly what I'd worried about all along. For once, my crazy ass parental paranoia was right! In that moment, I wasn't me; I wasn't Jenny, former classmate. I wasn't a writer, event planner, or even a person.

To them, I was Mom, and that's all. I was having a *Pretty Woman* moment, only, y'know, less hookery, and more minivan mafia. They saw one thing and one thing only. Julia Roberts wouldn't stand for this shit! Some people hear what you do, what your "job" is, or how you devote the majority of your time, and in their minds, it becomes all that you are, especially when it comes to jobs as . . . *serious* . . . as trolling the red-light district or raising children. As Hostest with the Mostest, I had to keep a smile on my face, but believe you me, I wanted to put their asses in time out.

There was no use fighting it once I showed up to the farewell breakfast the next morning. The attendees looked at me as though they'd seen a fucking ghost because they honestly thought I would have perished over the course of the night from alcohol poisoning. I just smiled like I had at the reunion and laughed at the jokes about how "drunk" I was the previous night and how hungover I must be. Really, I was thinking, "Bitch! That's just who I am!"

Make a child with your genitals and suddenly the world thinks you should be wearing turtlenecks and discussing laundry detergent. I'll do the electric slide if I fucking want to! *With* a drink in my hand! *Without* spilling! Stick that in your sippy cup and suck it! The trash might go out more than I do, but at least, unlike my classmates, my maturity level has changed. That's right—it went *down*. I'm even *less* mature now! Kiss my ass, ya bunch of turds! What?? What do you expect from someone trapped at home with whacked-out little kids all day every day?

CHAPTER **15**

THANK THE SWEET GRILLED CHEEZUS FOR CANCELED PLANS

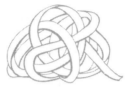

DESPITE MY SHORT STINT AS Julia Roberts, I marked down my ten-year reunion as a good time. Beggars can't be choosers, and I had begged my ass off for the chance to spend two hours without being asked for food while peeing, or hearing the sound of an entire bin of toys being dumped onto my newly cleaned living room floor. As much as I relish those fleeting and rare chances to get out of the house (because at least once a week it feels like the walls of this house are closing in on me and if I don't leave the confines of this place I will scream) even though my kids usually have to tag along, it is a pain in the ass to even walk out of the front door into the real world.

I long for the days when all I had to worry about before leaving the house was how my ass looked in my skin-tight pants or super short-shorts (because I could wear those back then without worrying about educating the world on where babies *really* come from via visual aid) and if my makeup looked decent. I want to slap the shit out of old (young) me. I didn't even *need* makeup! I should have taken advantage of that crap while I had the chance. These days, I'd bathe myself in anti-wrinkle cream if I could. I'd let Buffalo Bill put me in the damn hole if it meant a never-ending supply of hydrating lotion!

73

To get out of the house now is like a production of *Les Miserables*—an impossible amount of acts that feel like they may never end, extreme dramatics, unflattering costumes, and being concerned that I look like a cheap hooker. Not even Julia as Vivian Ward was a *cheap* hooker! As much of a martini sipping Hot Mom as I long to be, I'm a grown ass woman with two kids. There is no excuse to look like a bargain prostitute. By the end of just making myself presentable, I'm so damn worn out that all I want to do is go to bed. Bed is awesome.

Getting myself ready to go is not even the most time-consuming task, believe it or not. Whether the kids are coming with me or staying at home with whomever I could con into thinking they behave like actual humans and not rabid cavemen (and this is typically a one shot deal. No one has ever agreed to come back more than once!) putting together and preparing the insane multitude of shit they will need while we are out or I am gone is a task that I believe may inspire a bald trend. I've never had a stronger desire to tear my frickin' hair out strand by strand as I have due to the high level of worry that occurs about forgetting what I think are important things for the kids.

Not packing enough of the "right" thing. Will they eat, and will it be enough? What if they get sick or fall and get hurt and call for me? What if they screech that they want to go home in the middle of a crowded public place and ruin everyone else's fun time and some judgy old twat decides to try to school me on how to parent the "right" way? Do I need to bring extra clothes just in case of an accident? How about nap time? We can't possibly jeopardize nap time! What if they don't miss me at all??

The mind—it never quits. It is full of these miniscule worries that slowly drive us bananas over the course of the outing. It can't remember why the hell I walked into the living room, but it can't seem to leave me alone about the

Tupperware of Cheez-Its I accidentally left on the kitchen counter. Even if I successfully avoided looking like a five-dollar prostitute on half-off Hump Day, I have now effectively mentally beaten the piss out of myself. It is hard to hide the look of exhaustion to the point of insanity. All this manual labor to get myself the out of this God-forsaken house before I run away and join the sideshow (I'd say circus, but that would mean I'd have to spend more time surrounded by kids. No thanks.), since that's the only place that would take me looking as crazy as I usually do at times like these, and I begin to wonder if going out is even worth it at all?

If I take them along, they will bitch, moan, and complain the entire time about stupid nonsensical bullshit like "my legs are *allergic* to walking!" or how they'd rather be doing something fun like playing at Chuck-E-Cheese's (a.k.a. the seventh circle of Hell) beating you with a plastic hammer in the brain. No, not literally! My kids are assholes, not violent psychopaths. Most of the time. If I *leave* them, as much as they annoy the ever-loving piss out of me, I will miss them the *entire* time and want to go home.

Even if I know for certain that I have all of the bases covered, everything taken care of and provided for, just in case (even the extremely paranoid worry crap), I still cannot manage to relax. I'd blame my vagina for never letting me forget the hell I put it through, but I think it's just me. It just comes with the territory of having kids. There is simply no winning this one! Or at least, that's what I *thought*.

There, underneath my reclusive Don't Call Me Mom rock I'd only peeked out of long enough to yet again be pigeonholed by stereotypical crap, attempting to avoid the real world so I wouldn't drop-kick anyone in their baby-maker out of frustration, it came. A magical occasion every parent should be thankful for. Like a break in the clouds on a day where you thought the sky would never stop pissing on you, the sun comes through and shines down right onto your face. You smile, close your eyes, and look up to the sky with your arms outstretched like those bitches in all the tampon commercials, while fat little cherubs sing and unicorns are farting rainbows and prancing around you. It's the call to tell you the plans you've been freaking your shit out about for the last twenty-four hours straight have been *cancelled*! It felt like pooping after being constipated for a week; pure unadulterated bliss.

Perhaps this is one of those times where I should take a step back to look at my life as a whole and maybe think, *Is this what madness feels like?* I can't exactly be sure, what with the kids leeching off my few remaining brain cells at all times, but if I had to make a wager, it would be madness. I guess Half-off Hooker Hump Day will have to find a new lady of the night, because this ass will be parked comfortably on my couch, binge-watching Netflix.

CHAPTER **16**

ONE BIN OF BABY SHIT AWAY FROM AN EPISODE OF HOARDERS

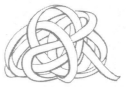

I DIDN'T TELL MANY PEOPLE about my apprehension and resistance to the term *mom* and everything I thought it stood for. Come to think of it, I didn't tell anyone. I didn't think anyone would be able to understand this odd situation when I didn't really understand it myself. I've always been a chronic over-thinker, to my own detriment, so I figured my friends' responses would all be the same.

Oh, it'll fall into place!

Don't worry!

It'll come naturally!

Ugh. Barf. No thanks. None of that felt as real as what I was feeling.

While the cynic in me thinks most people who dole out parenting advice on the fly are know-it-all asshats just trying to convince themselves their own choices are the right ones, I know my friends would have tried to make me feel better. But there's nothing natural about wiping a shitty little butt while it's still pooping (why do they do that???) or months—sometimes even years—of sleep deprivation. It would only serve to make me feel worse to hear that it's all supposed to come naturally, and then, it doesn't. Maybe I'm being too negative. Maybe I should swallow my pride, accept the advice, hold my head up high, and trudge through the waist-high bullshit until it feels right! Then again, my mom always told me that my boobs would eventually come naturally, and *that* never happened—so why should I believe that one day this whole "motherhood" thing would?

The only thing to do during the times I'm feeling like I'm sitting atop the Worst Mom Ever float in the Terrible Parents Parade is go shopping. (It's true and you damn well know it!) Look—there's nothing like a little bit of retail therapy to perk up the soul. Unless it's bathing suit shopping. Or really any kind of shopping where I have to try something on that I swear is my size and it ain't. Not cool, hips. Foul play, there! Mental anguish-free shopping truly only comes in one form: kids' clothes. Even for someone *else's* kid; there's not much better than squee-ing about teensy adorable this and thats.

Even though I don't want to, I have to go ahead and feed into stereotypes about women and say that I *love* to shop. Clothes, decorations, shit I don't really need but my brain insists I have to have—anything but groceries. I love browsing through rack after rack and bringing home new things to cram into my house—even better if what I bought was on sale. I love shopping so damn much that there are times I actually take pleasure in hearing the kids whine about how they absolutely cannot walk even one more step or they will collapse. You're *five*. Your legs are basically brand new. Get the fuck over it.

Regardless of the whining, complaining, or harsh, unforgiving overhead lighting, my love for shopping is an unbreakable bond, much to my husband's dismay. Shopping is my legal drug that should probably be illegal. With all that said, one would think that having kids would really work out in my favor because those little f'ers grow so damn fast they require *constant* shopping! It should be like Heaven on Earth for me, the cracked-out shopping fiend. Thomas can't even bitch about it because it's a need and not a want, unlike ransacking the cardigans at Target for myself. Acceptable frequent clothes shopping trips? What could possibly be bad about that? Not to mention the fact that you never have to worry about having one of those petrifying "Holy shit! Where did that patch of cellulite come from?" moments in the fitting room surrounded by funhouse mirrors. Kids look good in everything. Buncha assholes.

It came as a shock to me the day I realized this was actually my worst nightmare camouflaged by cutesy designs and teeny tiny t-shirts with infuriating little snaps. I never should have challenged my damn uterus. After spending hours skipping through aisles of clothing stores, more "awwww!"s than I can count, and blowing a bunch of money on "just the most *adorable* things I have ever seen!!" without feeling even a gram of guilt about it, I had to come home and put these treasures in their specific places. I must block this part out every single time it happens. I guess it's also possible that I get so high from the rush of shopping that reality slips away into the abyss of nothing that is now my brain. Fact is, buying new clothes for kids can only mean a few things: either they have ruined what you bought them because they are destructive monsters who won't stop scooting across the carpet like dogs with itchy buttholes, or they have grown.

Kids grow up! Why the hell didn't anyone tell me this??

These frequent fun-filled clothes shopping trips I was going on meant that my babies were growing, and *fast*. Frequent kiddie-clothes shopping trips mean that, before you know it, your adorable little baby in the adorable little clothes with the adorable little designs (and infuriating snaps) won't be a baby for very much longer; maybe they already aren't a baby anymore and you missed it! Maybe you are completely in denial and still shoving them into a tiny onesie like an overstuffed sausage . . . not that I'd know from experience or anything. I really feel like I should be able to file a complaint about this. This is not okay.

Back-to-school shopping is the absolute worst. I come home in a blissful buzz with bags upon bags full of new clothes with which I will force my child to wear, and then proceeded to skip into their bedrooms, open their drawers, and there they are . . . staring me in the face. The clothes I had skipped home with from my *last* kiddie-clothes shopping excursion. The clothes that no longer fit, which is why I went shopping in the first place. The clothes that now need to be replaced with these new clothes that just five minutes before I had been excited about, but now loathe with every fiber of my being. The clothes that are too small because my baby is too big. My *baby*! The fuck?

What could and *should* be a ninety-second process of scooping out the old stuff, tossing it in a box, and neatly putting the new stuff in its place becomes an hour long beat down of my heart. Each time I pull open one of those drawers with the intention of filling it with larger sized clothes, the wind gets knocked out of me and I have to take a seat. Once I sit down and, one by one, pull out the clothes that once fit but are now too small for my baby, who is really not so much a baby, I die a little inside.

One by one I stare at them, remembering each time my not-so baby wore it. I remember how cute they were, how it got a little stain that took forever to come out, but I just loved *this* onesie or *that* teeny tiny pair of pants so much that the thought of my will-always-be-my-baby not wearing it anymore made me sad. Not the "damn my milk is gone and I still have an Oreo left to dip" kind of sad, but the kind of sad you feel when you go to a Waffle House because you've been craving ginormous Belgian waffles smothered in butter and syrup for an entire week, and you *totally* deserve it because you've been eating super healthy for like, a day, only to get there and have them tell you they're all out. A *waffle* place is out of waffles. How in the hell does that happen?

My kids acted like the entire fucking world was crumbling when that happened not so long ago, and those red faces, crumpled lips, and long runny booger trails reminded me of exactly how I feel while cleaning out their drawers. Why do bad things happen to good people? Can't we just cryogenically freeze our kids to keep them teeny tiny forever? No? That would be bad? Ugh. It's just not fair!

One day you have drawers stuffed full of the tiniest onesies and the most precious socks you have ever seen, and then in the blink of an eye, you're clearing out the very last of the clothing marked TODDLER and in tramples the BOYS or GIRLS size small. Not newborn, no months on the tags or weight scales to choose from; not even an uppercase T. Where in the flying fart did your baby go? And how did you miss this transition? Shouldn't there have been some kind of parade or alarm? Maybe a smoke signal? Bullhorn to the eardrum? Screw you, people who said "they grow up too fast"! I refuse to acknowledge that you were right!

This predicament has proven to be such a horrific experience that I have to confess something right now. It's been weighing on me for a very long time and I just don't think I can continue without getting this off of my chest: I stopped getting rid of the clothes altogether. I can't bear to part with them. I haven't been able to in *years*.

My *baby* had his first diarrhea blow out in that onesie! How can I let that go?? But . . . it says Stud Muffin on it and he ate his first ice cream cone while he was wearing this one! How can I possibly get rid of it? Me, the woman who 9 times out of 10 can't remember what I had for dinner last night, can recall ridiculous details about specific days my children wore specific clothing years ago. I have a problem.

How can I get rid of it, I ask again? The answer is: I can't. I'm weak. I'm weak and, damnit, I am sentimental! First the waterworks, and now this? Does it ever end? Since we're on this whole "confession" thing, I suppose it's only right to also admit that sentimentality and the inability to accept that my children are growing up aren't the *only* reasons I can't let go of baby clothes. You see, the last time I decided I was finally ready to purge all the baby shit I had sitting around no longer being used because my stupid baby decided to grow up on me without asking permission, I found myself knocked up a week later. To add insult to injury, we would soon find out I was pregnant with the same gender we already had. We could have used all of those clothes! This only made me bitter and too terrified of the consequences to let anything go ever again. I am convinced that the moment you sell, donate, or give away the very last of the baby clothes, your uterus starts giggling like a maniac and decides to stick a knife in your back by filling itself with fetus.

Thomas is absolutely no help whatsoever, because he always comes moseying out of one of the kids' rooms after I have delegated the task of clothes sorting to him, and holds something ridiculously darling and asks me, "Does this still fit?" The answer is no, but I tell him yes. Do not dangle these things in my face and then expect me to be able to let them go! Who do you think I am? I want you to go through these things because I can't do it myself without going crazy, dumbass!!

I'm sorry! I love you!

If I were the eternally optimistic type, I might have been able to see this as just more of an excuse to shop, but I know better. I know that this brings you right back to square one. There you are with a cornucopia of baby clothes and no baby to put them in anymore. Not even the baby you insist is still your baby but is actually forty years old. You might even find yourself bribing said forty-year-old baby to try on a onesie, just for old time's sake.

Currently, a giant Tupperware tub lies at the foot of my bed. A giant Tupperware tub full of baby clothes. A giant Tupperware tub full of baby clothes that I absolutely refuse to get rid of, not only because I am emotionally attached to every single stupid article of clothing in it, but because I am convinced that the moment I do, I will yet again find myself pregnant. No vacancy! The tub at the end of my bed is overflowing. It's actually a little embarrassing to look at, yet still, I can't part with it. Or the tub in Parker's closet. Or the two tubs in Holden's. Or with the five tubs in the garage.

I *definitely* have a problem. I'm afraid Thomas is going to take secret video of the inside of our house and submit it to *Hoarders*, begging for help because his wife has mental issues and an unhealthy attachment to tiny poo-stained pants.

My new reality: cleaning out my kids' drawers nearly triggers an emotional breakdown. My memory might be shot, but I'm pretty sure I didn't agree to this.

And now I want waffles.

CHAPTER 17

WHY ALL PARENTS DESERVE A FRICKIN' OSCAR

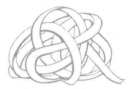

IT ALWAYS STRUCK ME AS odd on Christmas morning when my Dad would open gifts that were labeled To: Dad, From: Santa. Of course, at first, I totally bought the ruse. *Wow! Daddy must have been good this year! That sure is an expensive toy!* Once that tender age of gullibility faded, and I knew that Santa was as real as Christina Aguilera's boobs, the truth smacked me in the face like a wet blanket. I still didn't completely get it, though. Why is my dad not only buying himself shit, but wrapping it up, putting it under the tree, and opening it like he didn't already know what it was? What a frickin' weirdo!

Becoming a "responsible adult" sucked ass because it quickly dawned on me why my dad was so "weird," or maybe I should say, why he *wasn't*. No more presents! At least, not like when I was little and my parents had the pleasure of tricking me by swearing they didn't get me what I wanted. I'd spend weeks thinking I had the worst parents *ever*, only to find my dream present under the tree on Christmas morning. In the "awesomeness" (read: suckassery) we refer to as adulthood, if I wanted something, I had to buy it myself. No one else was going to. So, *that's* what my dad was up to all those years! He bought everyone else all the crap they wanted, but no one ever really got *him* anything.

If we did, it was with his own money. Ew. Why *not* go out and get exactly what he wanted for himself instead of just settling for yet another heinous Christmas sweater or billionth hideous festive tie?

It's a scientific fact that no matter how old you get, you will *always* love tearing into fresh wrapping paper; that is the full-on truth. I don't have any studies to back this up, but I am pretty damn sure there's no arguing to be done here. Responsible adulthood seemed so . . . *sad*. Where did all of the mystery, intrigue, and surprises go? Is that how parenthood is? Is my Dad who *I* am destined to become? Would I resort to Christmas shopping for myself to avoid getting ties covered in candy canes and elves? How could I *not* wonder? To: him From: him presents aside, my dad always seemed so surprised and happy when I brought home some handmade junk, or cheesy store-bought piece of crap for him, even though he probably already knew all about it. Hello? Credit card statements, anyone? Was it an act? Did he know? Did the guy who very early on in my life was dubbed "the man who has everything" hate the junk I gave him? As a child, I never really thought about it. He acted like he loved it, so he must have loved it! I'm an awesome gift-giver—and at such a young age? I must have been a child prodigy!

So many questions bouncing around in my head that, of course, were quickly forgotten and replaced with something like the lyrics to "MMMBop," or Leonardo DiCaprio's favorite vegetables. Priorities, man.

The week before Christmas of Holden's first year of school was exciting to me for one reason only (which is the same reason every holiday that year had been exciting thus far): he would finally be making me gifts that I wouldn't have to con him into making myself. *Real* gifts. I didn't really care what they were, just that I was finally not involved in the preparation or choosing of them. In "like father like son-in-law" fashion, Thomas had to provide the money for Holden to go shopping for us. His school's PTA had set up a little gift shop for the students, separated into sections like "for mom," "for dad," "for grandpa," so on and so forth. It made the process really easy for dense little kids who, without guidance, would bring mommy home a jockstrap or beard-blaster shaving cream. Talk about the making of awkward PTA meetings.

It had been a long ass time since I'd felt so excited about *any* holiday season—since I was a kid myself, now that I think about it. Grinchy old me couldn't wait to see what he got me come Christmas morning—even if he bought it with my money. I packed the cash we'd set aside for Holden to spend on each of us into his book bag and carted him off to school. In my head, I was thinking back to when I used to go shopping for *my* parents and how awesome I felt getting that sucker gift wrapped, and being able to come home and put something *I* picked out and bought for someone else under the tree for the first time; how fantastic it was to be the only one who knew what that gift was. The roles had finally changed, and soon I'd get to see Holden's selection all wrapped up. I was beyond excited for the anticipation to kill me, and to see him looking so pleased with himself that he had a secret that was all his own. And wrapping paper! Let me at it!

He came home from school that afternoon with an enormously proud look upon his face, plopped down his backpack onto the kitchen table, and yanked out a plastic grocery bag. "Look what I got!" he exclaimed, rummaging through the bag's contents. I wandered over to him, expecting history to have repeated itself and for all of his gifts to be wrapped already, when Holden found what he was looking for and yanked it out in broad daylight.

"This is what I got for *you*, Mommy!"

By the time I realized what he had said, it was too late. I'd seen the gift. It was the most horrendous Pepto Bismol pink keychain I'd ever laid eyes on, and dangling from it was a shiny, silver *"#1 Mom!"* charm. Like a vampire hit by daylight and a cross covered in garlic, I threw my arms in front of my face and screamed for the child to hide it from me. *I* knew the damage had already been done, but it didn't need to be ruined for him, too.

When the time came to finally open my gift on Christmas morning, I could tell by the pee-pee-like dance Holden was doing that he was eager for me to open his gift. Even though I knew what I'd be opening; even though I'd already seen it and was well aware that it was the gaudiest piece of junk on the planet, it didn't matter. Not one bit. Big, wide, shocked eyes—gasping and over-the-top Scarlett O'Hara type dramatics—to any adult it would be extremely obvious that I was totally full of shit and putting on a poorly acted show, but to Holden, that heinous thing was the most amazing gift I had ever received. He was so proud of himself for picking out something I "loved." Immediately, I attached it to my key-ring, and any and every time we had to go somewhere, I made a huge deal out of it just because it made him happy, which made *me* happy. Even if it was hideous. No, seriously; it was *hideous*.

Poor Thomas had to do the same thing when he opened his gift: an ink pen that said "I love grandpa."

Who the hell was running that gift shop?? Put down the crack pipe, PTA Pam! But hey, at least he was surprised!

The funny thing is, that ugly little keychain really did prove to be a total piece of junk. It only took about a month for it to break, get lost, and was never seen again. No longer did my keys scream in bright pink letters that I am the "#1 Mom!" and while I should have been relieved, I was actually teary-eyed when I realized it was really gone. My *baby* gave me that! It was a very sad time, but come Mother's Day, I was *helping* to hide my own presents. The kids still totally bought my "surprised" performances, which led me to believe that I should be winning Oscars. I *must* be good if even *I* can forget where I hid something, and then end up genuinely surprised once it's been discovered a month later behind a chair and I finally receive it. Watch the hell out, Meryl Streep, I'm coming for your shiny bald trophy!

Or . . . maybe all of that is just the lovely side effect of the dreaded mommy-brain.

My parents had boxes of mine and my brother's elementary school drawings and crafting atrocities stored in our family home's pantry, the attic, and really anywhere with extra space. I always thought it was strange to hang onto a random sheet of construction paper with a stick figure drawn with crayon until that Christmas with Holden. It doesn't matter how awful or nonsensical a drawing is or how poorly something is spelled. It doesn't even matter if it's just a bunch of scribbles on a piece of dirty ass paper. I don't care if one of my brats doodles a picture of me with a manly beast-like five o'clock shadow for Christmas and then follows it up with a can of beard-blasting shaving cream from the PTA crack house gift booth for my birthday. I might develop some sort of extreme complex about my skin and end up spending a small fortune on laser hair removal . . . but I'd still love every second of it.

Why?

Because it came from *them*—my babies! Because they love me enough to take the time to give or make something just for me.

And because they're dumb little kids and don't know any better. I know, I still think it's totally strange. The only thing I wouldn't love is a booger wiped on a piece of paper and handed to me while still wet—but at least it wasn't wiped on the couch! It was moments like these when I started to worry about myself and just how much my brain was being melted by whining and the infernal yellow square the kids loved so much. I shouldn't think about it; the truth is a scary mo-fo.

From now on, I think "Santa" is going to reward me for being such a good girl. Don't ever tell him I said so, but maybe, *just* maybe, Dad had the right idea. Blame it on Santa! Mama needs a new pair of shoes!

CHAPTER 18

LOOK, MA! I CAN PEE AND BRUSH MY TEETH AT THE SAME TIME! AND OTHER TERRIBLE IDEAS

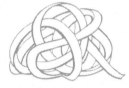

THE RELIEF EXPERIENCED ONCE ALL the holidays have passed is one that cannot be described with words—especially if you have kids. No more crowds, no more crazy shopping, no more bargain hunting; at last, a break! Wrong. There is never a break with kids. The holidays actually knock you right off your game. Be aware! Settling back into real life is a real bitch. There's no more magic to threaten the young'uns with. You have to resort to good ol' fashioned resourcefulness. It comes in the form of something *so* simple, something you might never expect: multi-tasking.

This is one of the most useful skills ever when it comes to raising children, other than an insane amount of patience and the ability to function on less than three hours of consecutive sleep for months on end. It is a skill that is utilized every single moment of every single day without even realizing it because when it comes to kids, doing one thing at a time is simply impossible. Many days, you realize as you pour a bowl of cereal for yourself at 1 p.m. that you never got around to actually eating a real breakfast. Where the hell did the day go?

The first few years of parenthood are like being blackout sorority girl wasted. You stumble around, completely disoriented and incoherent, can't account for the previous three hours of your life, and have *no* clue why you are so sticky or how the kitchen got completely destroyed. Many mornings, you awake from a strangely deep slumber wondering how in the hell did all of these people get in my bed? And *when*? At least in the case of parenthood, you don't question your morals or standards, but most definitely your sanity. Somehow, you know that if you are going to survive the next eighteen or so years and come out the other end without booking an extended stay at the nut-farm, things have to change.

From just witnessing how absolutely insane other people's kids are in public, I once looked at my brand new sleeping newborn and of *course* swore he would be easier. Those first few days, or maybe even first few hours of being a parent, are full of self-delusion due to wonderfully sweet impossibilities and that new baby smell. You know the one. That "new baby" smell will get you drunk quicker than moonshine! It will convince you that you should have more babies as soon as possible, and that you have the strength to lift a car off the ground like Superman. You are not Superman. You are tired and delusional. Let that first projectile-poo hit you and come on back down to earth.

Obviously, multitasking isn't anything *new* we parents have to learn. It's been around since the dawn of time. It's something we've been doing our entire lives because most of us are born with the "work smarter, not harder" gene deep down inside, annoying the piss out of us every time we try to procrastinate. Even if we *never* work smarter, that tiny obnoxious voice in our heads screams that we should be. As babies, it's as simple as blinking and breathing, and then we move on to bigger and better things like clapping our hands and "singing" at the same time. I use the term *singing* very loosely, but it counts.

Even earlier—we *must* learn to breathe while we drink from a boob or bottle—that *totally* counts. Multitasking is the *first* thing we ever learn to do. Writing and talking at the same time totally came in handy at school. Homework while watching TV? It was an absolute must due to not having DVR back in my day (Yeah. I admitted it. I'm old. Deal with it!) and a limited supply of VHS tapes to record onto. I truly don't know what young me would have done without multitasking. *Dawson's Creek* certainly wasn't going to watch itself!

If my parents could walk uphill both ways to school in the snow with no shoes and a broken leg, I'm sure that *somehow* I would have managed, though.

Never did I like to describe my early days of motherhood as "busy" because I wasn't running around to appointments, spending hours at the grocery store, or going on buttloads of mind-numbing errands, but they were most definitely full. A standard day consisted of getting both kids up, fed, and ready for the day. I made sure Holden's lunch was packed, his book bag was ready, and then dropped him off at school on time. Usually, I would then attempt to work off some of this excess flab I was still refusing to refer to as anything other than "baby weight" while trying to entertain a toddler who thought riding the dog like a horse around the house was the most awesome shit ever. The dog disagreed wholeheartedly.

Before I knew it, it was lunch time, then nap time, then wake up toddler and get screamed at time. From there, we rushed to school pickup, which is a damn nightmare because half the population has no idea how to drive, let alone park. I'm looking at you, minivan mafia mom! After that, it was parental torture, a.k.a. homework time, then toss the kids outside so they don't convince me trading them to the Gypsies is a stellar idea time, and then back in to shove a snack into them and start making dinner. As if that wasn't enough—praise the stars in the sky—then comes bath and *bed* time . . . only to wake up and do it all over again. And people wonder why I say that I've lost my fucking mind.

As much as monotony can make one feel like Jack Nicholson in *The Shining*, this routine worked for us. We had it down to a science. Any deviation from this routine and the entire day would go to shit. I know; what a stick in the mud I was! What about excitement and spontaneity? That nonsense can wait for the weekends!

Not long into Holden's kindergarten year, I became convinced the public school system was designed to torture parents, what with confusing ass homework that we have to help with. We had been so excited when school ended for us because we *thought* it meant we'd never have to do homework or attempt the utter horseshit that is algebra ever again. Then the elementary school here just *had* to go and toss in a half day, just for good measure. *Every* Wednesday of Holden's first year in school. Not cool. There went my routine, floating right out the window. Our little lunch-nap-scream dance that we had perfected for months poofed into thin air. Wednesdays were whores. Dirty, ball-licking whores. Because of that one little switch up that might have seemed so miniscule to the outside world, the house devolved into utter chaos. Moments like those—where you're ready to request a pretty white jacket that straps in the back because life has gone absolutely batshit crazy and you barely have time to breathe—are ones in which parents must remind themselves that white padded rooms *sound* fun, but would get old fast.

People used to tell me I was "lucky" to have a three-year-old who still napped, but they don't realize that this scheduled "luck" came with a very steep price. If that threenager didn't get this nap he so graciously blessed us with, and for an adequate amount of time, he would go full-on invasion of the body-snatchers pod person, or as I lovingly refer to it: Attack of the Poddler. If you bore witness to this, you would swear the only remedy to the situation would be to call a young priest and an old priest and bless a tub full of water. In short—the child *had* to have this nap! Which in turn meant I *had* to make this nap happen at all costs if I didn't want beds levitating and split pea soup spewed all over me.

Wednesdays didn't just muck up the schedule; they were downright *dangerous* to my health. Probably everyone else within a five-mile radius of our house, as well.

It was, and still always is, a major pain in the butthole to get to the school, fight other parents for a coveted parking spot (that is what my life has come to), wait for the kid to be released, and then make it home in a reasonable amount of time. Hold onto your ass if you show up five minutes late (and by late I actually mean early); the minivan mafia will eat you alive. They are *brutal*. It's worse than the mall on Christmas Eve; and if it's raining? Fucking fogeddaboutit!

I just so happened to be that lucky one day, and by the time we got home, I was drenched in stanky panic sweat, and Parker was bordering on a demonic possession level of crankiness. Drastic measures needed to be taken to keep the beast at bay. There had been no time to pee during all of the madness, so for the previous forty-five minutes, I'd been holding it. Let's be very honest here—for a mom who vaginally gave birth to two children in two years, forty-five minutes is an eternity. My bladder was *screaming*. Someone call Guinness! Bring on the man in a suit with his fancy stopwatch to time this shit!

I shoved the children through our house's threshold and forced their little asses up the stairs. While doing the pee-pee dance, I managed to get toothpaste on their toothbrushes, but my poor beat-up bladder just couldn't hold it anymore. I ripped down my pants and I plopped faster than I have ever plopped before, just thankful that none of my stream missed the toilet. Parker likes to feign independence, and will insist upon doing things far beyond his ability, but tooth brushing just isn't one of them. I'd forgotten about that in my urine rush. He picked up his toothbrush and walked over to me while I was still unleashing what I swear was the longest pee of my life, and said, "Mommy! I need help!" Without even a second thought and/or a care in the world—because it was late and we were out of time—with the multitasking Gods as my witnesses . . . I began brushing his teeth with my pants around my ankles and pee pouring out of me. I got that kid down for a nap before the ground opened up and demons started roaming the earth too. I consider that a *major* win.

My life as a parent was now officially one lived with absolutely no shame and a strong forcefield against embarrassment . . . for the most part. *And* it was one lived with a prison-bitch-type relationship with multitasking; me being the bottom here. I had to contemplate if perhaps I suffered from Stockholm syndrome because I truly considered multitasking to be my lifesaver. (The hard kind, though. The chewy ones are frickin' *nasty*.) What the hell happened to me? Should I have felt shame? Embarrassment? Acceptance? It was an odd feeling, but one I knew deep down I needed to get used to. I am not a fan of this whole "reality" thing.

Multitasking was mom-me's BFF. Or maybe it was more like a frenemy; someone/thing you keep close because if you push them away, they will attack like a rabid dog. Multitasking is my Regina George; the meanest of the mean girls. I loved it, but it repeatedly kicked my ass. It must be *some* kind of mind control, because somehow I got to the point where I began allowing family members to poop in the bathroom while I took a shower, just to save time . . . but maybe that has more to do with true love. You *have* to love someone to allow something like that.

True love is taking a shower, only to open the curtain and get covered in someone else's cloud of fresh colon cologne . . . or maybe you just love the smell of rectal vomit, in which case, you should seek help.

CHAPTER 19

A MOM WOULDN'T KNOW SILENCE IF IT CRAPPED IN ITS HANDS AND CLAPPED IN HER FACE!

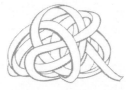

THERE'S NO PRETENDING HERE; I had absolutely no idea what the hell I was doing anymore. I wouldn't exactly call it an identity crisis, but I had questions. The fibbing, the simultaneous peeing and tooth brushing—was I doing the right thing? Making the right choices? No one could ever answer that. I knew my kids were *my* kids, and at the end of the day, I knew them better than anyone else, but sometimes I just wanted a clear cut yes or no instead of having to figure it all out for myself. *And* I wanted the truth—not this sugar-coated BS that people float out into the atmosphere that makes those of us just keeping our heads above water feel like just letting ourselves drown.

People are totally into giving their opinions until you actually ask for it—and I mean REAL advice, not the "I'm the best parent ever and you suck old saggy balls" condescending kind. Once you *ask* for real, truthful, non-judgy help, you get crickets. Well, not exactly. There was *always* noise, just not the noise I was looking for.

If I were ever greeted by the sound of silence, I wouldn't know what the hell it was. During any given point on any given day, someone was banging on something, throwing something, whining that something was being thrown, or that they want something but it was taken from them. It is *always* something. *Always.* I wouldn't even know silence if it crept up behind me and started furiously dry humping my leg. In my head, I imagine that silence would be terribly frightening. Mostly because I know that the sound of silence in a house with a child occupant means that something is being destroyed, being used to destroy, smashed into something, or flushed down the toilet. My kids would *never* use what I can only assume is wizard magic to silently body-slam a lamp and snap it in half for the third time or hide turds in their closets. I've only been *told* that this whole mysterious "silence" thing I keep hearing (or not hearing) about should be very, very suspicious.

To drown out the constant chorus of somethings, I started to talk to myself. This does not make me crazy—it makes me *crafty*. There is a difference. How else would I keep my conversational skills sharp? Okay, maybe not *sharp*, but better than babbling baby talk. When I would run out of things to say to myself—which happened often since I'm not that much of a talker to someone who doesn't respond—it would seem that I enjoyed singing a little song or humming a happy tune. Totally natural. Even those dwarves in *Snow White* whistled while they worked, so why not hum a little melody to drown out the madness that regularly swirls about in our heads and homes?

Personally, I attributed the loose grasp on the sanity I had left to my ability to be able to drown out small, annoying children yelling through empty toilet paper rolls like fucking megaphones by singing a little song. Loose is better than nothing! Any song would do. I have been known to sing ridiculously inappropriate lyrics to jams from my childhood, that in my naivety, were not awkward *at all* for eight-year-old me to be singing in the presence of other humans.

Countless times as an adult, I have heard songs I loved as a kid and been absolutely shocked now that I'm older and more aware, a.k.a. slightly less stupid, and finally understand the lyrics. Even still, I'll hum that shit around the kids. The little sanity it helped keep intact was worth it! It makes total sense! The sad truth of it is, though, that mindlessly singing Salt-N-Pepa's "Push It" (or some other inappropriate song. Frankie says "Relax" *might* be one of my old faithfuls) with the kids present is not my most disturbing musical offense, if you can believe it. I wish I could say it was a singular moment of weakness; that I caught myself, realized the error of my ways, and made a solemn vow never to repeat the same mistake again . . . but damnit, I'm human! People say the first step to recovery is to admit fault, so here goes nothing.

While washing the dishes one day with the kids shrieking at each other because their love/hate relationship was leaning more toward hate, I found myself in a bit of a dilemma. I was not quite ready to flip the bitch switch on them and go into full-on "mom" mode, complete with intimidating scowl (which took an extreme amount of practice, trust me), wagging finger, and booming voice of death. My hands were wet and covered in soap, and honestly, it just seemed like too much damn work to stop what I was doing to handle their asses. Plus, I really didn't like having to be mean ol' Mom. It didn't feel right. Sometimes it felt *good*, but still not quite right. Can't they just listen? Just once? Is that so much to ask?

Parenting advice may be obnoxious, but lemme tell ya, you really have to pick your battles wisely. That ability really comes in handy when dealing with children.

If you ask me, there is no sound on Earth more annoying than that of the small child whine. Not even nails on a chalkboard or the sound of a fork scraping across a plate can compare. The worst is being trapped in a car with it, but runner-up goes to hands stuck in a soapy sink full of dishes.

The way my logic worked was that if I stopped doing dishes before finishing, thus shutting the kids the hell up and stopping the coming of the apocalypse, I would still have to come back to the dishes, let the water get hot again, and try to get back into my scrubbing groove. That is far too many steps, and the kids should really learn to handle their own damn problems. I decided the best solution would be to keep my hands in the sink, scrub, and hum away the whining. Oh, and dance. Dancing is important. That way, I could shimmy my ass off while cleaning and keeping myself from snapping—win/win/win!

So hum I did, and I must say, the sound of running water along with the loud humming in my head really had a soothing effect on me. The only problem was that I now had that damn tune trapped in my brain like a worm; all day long I caught myself mindlessly humming it, tapping my foot to it, and backing it up like a dance party for one. It wasn't until one of the kids got so annoyed with me that they could no longer stand the sound of my voice, and demanded to know what and *why* I was humming constantly, that I decided it was time to evict my brain-worm. Why not share the internal happiness I was feeling with the creatures that caused me to be humming to drown them out in the first place? I took a little breath in, and then sang that shit out.

Imagine my shock and horror upon realizing that the euphoria and relief I'd given myself for the entire day was thanks to none other than the theme song to a certain popular preschool cartoon with a certain football head–shaped child who goes traipsing off with her stupid pet into places with dangerous wildlife. If you're a parent, you've likely been trapped watching this at least a handful of times, each time losing faith in humanity and regretting the choice to have children. Yes, that damn Dora again. I can't get away from her! I swear she's stalking me.

Blasphemy! It can't be!

But . . . I hate that song! I *hate* that show!

Just when I thought it couldn't possibly get any worse, the truth just *had* to dawn on me. The truth is a spiteful bitch.

Every tune I'd had stuck in my head for the past few years was not *anything* respectable, like a one-armed Def Leppard eighties hair band anthem, or the theatrical rendition of "Grease Lightning." It wasn't even the ever-popular fallback "Don't Stop Believing" of both past and recent Journey fame. Of course not.

I'd have been okay with nineties Britney Spears. Hell, I'd be just peachy with some Spice Girls platform-wearing "Girl Power!" pop stuck up there in my noggin, but no. It was *all* kiddie tunes; every last fucking one. How could something that brings me so much anger bring me so much happiness at the same time?

Oh, the humanity!

That obnoxious rascal and her oddly colored pet broke me without even breaking a sweat; without even appearing on my TV longer than it took me to change the channel in *years*!

What??? I have *some* integrity left! I have standards, people!

At least there is *one* perk to this infection of the brain that simply cannot be cured: my kids *hate* it when I sing their beloved shows' theme songs even more than I do. I am not ashamed to admit that it brings me great joy to torture them *so* fucking easily. We are a family, after all, and family suffers *together*!

I had no idea what was happening to me, but for the first time since procreating, I was pretty sure that, for the most part, I actually liked this whole "mom" thing. Ew.

CHAPTER **20**

IF YOU HAVEN'T MANHANDLED BABY POOP, YOU HAVEN'T LIVED

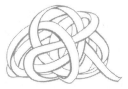

Beep beep beep beep!

The boys ran circles around the big open space in our living room in front of the fireplace. *Beep beep beep! Wooooo-wooooo!* They were both . . . firetrucks? Ambulances? Asshole Police cruisers? Annoying. That's what they were; annoying. I wondered if things might be different had my uterus produced female spawn instead of two penis wielders. I had been a dainty little girl, and any girl I might have would take after me, wouldn't they? On second thought . . . if I had a girl who took after me, she would be even louder, more disgusting, and far more annoying than my boys combined!

I am not, never have been, and probably never will be a "girly girl." Sure, I love makeup (I might even go as far as to say that I am having a clandestine affair with black eyeliner), but many days makeup is more of a necessity so I don't scare small children than a love of mine. I don't salivate over shoes or purses, and high fashion confuses the shit out of me. Really? You'd wear that? With that hair? But it looks like you have a penis on your head! I just don't get it. To be honest, I don't really want to. The day I think it's fashionable to wear a penis on my head is the day I'm crapping my adult diapers and can't eat solid foods. I'd probably be happy to even *see* a penis at that point.

This isn't some new development or phase in my life where I'm swearing off shaving and bras, thereby making people feel uncomfortable in public because my wild, bra-less nips are staring at them. I've always been this way. My mom was so excited to have a little girl she could dress up in pink frilly vomit, and instead had a child who perfectly defines of the term *tomboy*—me. Oops. The majority of my youth was spent climbing trees and swimming in the lake with the neighborhood boys even though I was repeatedly reminded that fish pooped in that water. In the time that was left once I'd made mud pies and played with worms, I would refuse to brush my hair until my brother would start calling me Rats Nest! My absolute *favorite* gross and un-girly thing to do above all else really took the cake, though: belching. Thank you to Christine at my eleventh birthday party sleepover for teaching me the fine art of the mega-belch after chugging bottles of Surge. Those were the days!

Ah, let's cut to the truth here: I *still* belch. And I'm damn good at it, too. I might not be able to climb trees in fear of breaking my back, and no way in *hell* am I swimming in a lake full of animal crap and creepy crawlies that could bite me or slither up into my hoo-ha, but I still feel totally awkward in dresses, and flip-flops are my go-to shoes. Even in the winter. Oh, and I pick my nose, too. I ain't ashamed!

None of my nasty, impolite, unladylike habits could have ever prepared me for the nasty that is children. *None.*

While I don't think anyone is ever completely prepared for the surprises, horrors, and joys the gift of parenthood keeps on giving, I didn't exactly think I was going in blind. I had TV, people; I watched it, a lot! Duh, poopy diapers and baby spit up! Not that I found the premise of being Head Butt-Wiper In Charge, constantly wiping excrement from someone else's ass all day long, to be appealing, but I just knew it came with the territory. You can't *not* know that, regardless of lack of experience. I truly didn't give much thought to how involved I would have to become with the bodily functions of other humans—*all* bodily functions. Neither did my husband. That would turn out to be a giant mistake—possibly a life-altering one.

I'm pretty sure when Thomas looks back at his experiences thus far on this journey called parenthood that we dove head first into, he'd prefer never to repeat a lot of stories to another living soul for as long as he lives. Actually, I wouldn't be the least bit surprised if he's blocked them from his own memory as to avoid large therapy bills. It's like Fight Club; you may know it has happened, but you *never* speak of it.

The man has been married to me for nearly a decade, so I would hope that he has learned by now that although he may never tell these stories, he can count on me doing so if it makes me giggle! He must spend a lot of his spare time clenching his ass cheeks in fear of what I'm going to say next. Thomas may have felt he was safe from this story ever being written for inquisitive eyes to read thanks to my deteriorating mommy-brain, and he could have gotten away with it if it weren't for that fateful day not so long ago when I sat in my living room, watching helplessly as the boys screeched and fought and destroyed everything in their paths.

Beep beep beep beep! Wooooooo-wooooo!

No matter how many times I used the dreaded and terrifying Mom Voice (we all know the one, complete with matching scowl) or threatened to sell the boys on Craigslist, they did not relent. This was one of those times that I could do nothing but wonder where I went wrong. Was it that second can of tuna I ate during pregnancy? The time I won Mom of the Year after Holden took a header off of the changing table? Was it the constant wishing I did while with child that both kids would have vaginas instead of penises? How did I get here? Why are the kids such a-holes? What am I doing? What am I *going* to do? What *is* the going rate for disobedient brats on the black market? Is this really my life? Do I have *any* control over it? It was then that the memory came flooding back to me. As awful as some things are, knowing you are not alone in these experiences gives one a little shred of hope that perhaps you haven't completely lost your mind, and maybe your child isn't out to destroy you after all. It does for me, anyway. That is why these stories *must* be told—whether Thomas likes it or not.

There's a reason we aren't given an instruction manual upon squeezing out new life and being shoved out of the hospital into the world to fend for ourselves. It's not because it doesn't exist, or that all babies are completely different, or any of that other crap people say. It's because if we were told what *really* happens after you take a baby home—the *truth* (if you strip away all that unconditional life-changing love crap) of the horrors you are about to behold . . . well, let's just say that the nutfarm would have far more residents, and there would be a lot more Little Orphan Annies singing for Daddy Warbucks. I kid . . . or do I?

A person of average intelligence doesn't need to crack open a baby book to know that one of the main job requirements to hold the title of "parent" is diaper changing. That same person of average intelligence understands that diaper changing includes a poopy nature. To continue with this whole "truth" thing—even without any experience— taking care of a child isn't rocket science. Baby crying? You'll automatically find yourself rocking back and forth, lightly patting whatever area your hand can reach, which is usually the butt, in the awkward and painfully uncomfortable position you've gotten yourself trapped in. (And it's *always* the most uncomfortable for you that is the most comfortable for them. Just ask my chronic back pain.) Baby hungry? Feed it! Baby bored? Toss a toy at it! Good baby! Easy baby! Piece of cake, right?

Hold on . . . let me stop laughing and catch my breath.

Despite the fact that eighties-nineties sitcoms made diaper changing look downright impossible and infuriating (and hilarious to us viewers), it's self-explanatory. They hit the nail on the head about nap times (if you get them at all) and bed times being a giant whore and accurately portrayed meal times as a loud and disgusting disaster of epic proportions. That's all well and good, but I found that the same frightening truths that knocked down the creation of an accurate baby instruction manual are the truths missing from these shows. It could have been an oversight, left on the cutting room floor by accident, but I smell a conspiracy.

No, really—I can *smell* it, and I'll tell you why.

We can blame the censors, or the critics, or the fact that networks just don't want their viewers barfing and then boycotting their channels, but where are the booger stories? A tale of parenthood cannot be accurate until you include at least one booger tale, and not just the runny kind that make snail trails down a kid's face. Please. Can we get real? The kind I'm referring to are the ones that are so big, you have to reach up your child's nose and pull those suckers out yourself. The kind that those booger-sucking bulb devices simply cannot handle. The kind you have to coax out carefully like a feral rabies-ridden animal hiding in a bush, and when you finally dislodge it from its lair, you are literally shocked a foot backwards because of its sheer mass.

How did something so big come out of something so little? And why am I inspecting it like it's an alien butt probe? And *why* is my kid screaming at me? They should be *thanking* me for removing something that *must* have been sitting on their brain and sucking out their life-force.

Unfortunately for me and fellow parents, boogers are not the worst of it. Oh no, we must cozy up to far more kinds of bodily excretions. Nose gremlins have become a cakewalk, all because of a four-syllable word that is only uttered in the confines of our own home; a word that instills fear into the hearts of grown men. That word, my friends, is *constipation*. Not just any stuffy-butted constipation, though. We're talking *baby* constipation.

Some may think other forms of poo are more formidable opponents of our gag reflex, such as the kind that gets smeared on bedroom walls like organic paint, or the lovely kind that takes liquid form and shoots across the room from a tiny ass-cannon, but I disagree wholeheartedly. You see, when both my boys were infants, they were plagued with reflux. Horrible, terrible, nasty thing that was. When you find a reflux medication that works, it's like the heavens opened up and here comes those fat naked cherubs again, floating around your head playing harps. It's a godsend. The beeping, fighting, and woo-wooing had *nothing* on being kept up all night by a screaming baby.

Finally, we could sleep at night because *they* could sleep at night, and the world was once again a bright and sunshiny place. This was not without consequence, though. In both cases, we had to learn through repeated experience. (What? It had been a while since Holden. Plenty of time for repeated brain bleachings before Parker came along and brought it all back up like burn-y stomach bile.) One occasion in particular, back when Holden was a fat-roll covered baby that tops them all. Not for me—I have my own horror stories—but for Thomas. Right now I bet he's wishing mom-brain had actually done its job, but he only has his own children to blame for jogging my memory!

It would appear that when you try to help a reflux baby keep from horking up the contents of their stomach, which sometimes consists of trying a bit of oatmeal or rice cereal in the bottles to do so (by recommendation of our pediatrician), not only does it keep the liquid down, but it *keeps* it down. Get what I'm hinting at here? Not too long after following the doctor's advice and dropping some oatmeal into every bottle, we noticed the puke decreasing. Rejoice! Confetti cannons! But wait . . . the poop was decreasing, too. Believe it or not, even after all the times I have been sharted on, I am a fan of poop. Pooping is good for you. A good poop can turn a bad day right around! *Not* pooping is just bad news for everyone. All babies do is eat, piss, shit, sleep (yes, I laughed while typing that), and cry, right? So what happens if you take one of those away?

Hell. *Hell* happens.

Baby Holden, who had finally been made happy thanks to the magic of reflux meds, had turned back into a red-faced, screaming, limb-thrashing demon baby. Like I said, *hell*. Even Satan himself would have been scared of Holden's ass.

We tried just about everything in the crap-ass excuse for a handbook we had (read: parenting book), and it all failed miserably, along with everything the pediatrician suggested once we called her at the end of our ropes. Prunes didn't work, even though everyone and their mother swore that would make his ass straight-up explode in no time flat. Pear juice? Fail. Some friends swore by laxative drops but the label said he wasn't old enough and we, being first time—a.k.a. horribly confused and overly-worried parents—never did anything a label told us not to do. I swear we thought some kind of alarm would sound if we *dared* to disobey. You know shit has gotten bad when you're crossing your fingers for an outbreak of airborne diarrhea.

There was really only one option left; one we'd been holding off on because the thought of implementing this form of relief was more than my weak stomach could handle. The pediatrician had suggested giving Holden a suppository. I kind of knew what it was, or I *thought* I did, anyway. Much to my horror, whatever vision I had in my head was wrong. So very, very wrong. A suppository wasn't an oral medication? What?? And you're telling me it has to be shoved *up his butt*? Seriously? And it has to *stay* there for five minutes even though the natural reaction will be to try and push it back out? Are you fucking *kidding* me? What is this, the friggin' Thunderdome? Two men enter, one turd leaves! Pretty damn sure the one to make it out alive would *not* be me!

Now that I knew a suppository was basically a butt-plug, I was yet again mistaken in thinking that I had a clear idea of what to expect. Things you put up your butt look just like the things you put in your mouth, only they go up your butt instead. This time I *knew* I had it right! No. Horrified moment number two (pun definitely intended) came when we opened the box and pulled out something that to me looked more like a hot glue stick than an aid to help grease a trapped turd. I took one look at that thing, had a mental vision of trying to force it up a tiny stuffed baby butthole, and felt my stomach turn over. It was not going to happen. Sorry, Thomas, this one's on you!

I'd say that he was pissed, but that would just be too obvious of a joke to make. Dude was *mad*. Not as mad as Holden, the un-pooper, but the kind of mad in cartoons where steam comically pours from the character's ears. Before you go thinking I am a cruel woman surely headed straight for divorce for making Thomas do this, you should know that I didn't leave the guy to go it alone. I stayed in the room at Holden's shoulders for moral support and to comfort him during the . . . delivery. Sound familiar? This kid was going to give birth to this turd if it was the last thing we did! Perhaps I should have considered this Thomas's penance for me being the one who had to blow my crotch out giving birth to the kid. You know what people say: revenge is a dish best served cold.

To spare everyone the horror, and what I am sure would be multiple sleepless nights coupled with a refusal to ever procreate, I will refrain from going into the gruesome details of what occurred in that room on that night so long ago, but because I think everyone deserves to know the truth that was kept from us, there are some things you must know.

1. No matter how small the baby, they can produce a turd the size of an adult. Not an adult turd, an *actual* adult. It doesn't seem physically possible, but once you see a tiny poop-chute turn inside out passing a lumberjack log, you can't unsee it.
2. Suppositories are a cruel and evil joke. And messy. Did I mention messy? The butt acts like a glue gun, melts the stick, and then squirts that junk right back out. But no poop.
3. By the time you're done with that pathetic failure of fecal Lamaze coaching, your kid has gone from pissed to hypersonic.

Not even I, the calm and comforting birthing coach, could soothe poor Holden. By this point, I think anyone in the same situation would be so exhausted, disturbed, and outrageously stressed out that they'd do just about *anything* to make it end, and I do mean *anything*.

This was where Thomas became the knight in shining armor. Wait, did I write shining? Definitely not shining, but he did the thing that no one else could do . . . or they *could* do, but definitely wouldn't. And by "they," I mean me. No fucking way. He went in like a surgeon and extracted that adult-sized log. By "extract," I mean *literally* used his bare hands and pulled the shit *out* of our child. My . . . hero? I didn't see this to confirm that it is actually what happened— above shoulder-level moral support only, remember? But considering the sound of a grown man screaming and the look-grimace-look-look away-look-grimace-look away thing I'd witnessed, I believed him. Even without the facial expressions and sound effects, the fact that he then washed his hands for a solid twenty minutes and appeared as though his life had been changed forever was proof enough. So much that I didn't let those hands come near me for a *very* long time. I didn't get taught to wipe front to back for nothin'. Get those poo-hands away from my lady junk!

Don't even start thinking that I should have rewarded him for a job well done. His reward is still letting him look at me after having my hoo-ha snipped twice and stitched back up bringing this giant turd-creating human into the world. I'll also never look at glue guns the same way again.

I think I just had an epiphany about why I refuse to craft. It all makes so much sense now!

For the past few years, I thought my cousin was just being a dick when he met Holden for the first time and said, "It all goes downhill from here," but now I'm thinking either he put some kind of voodoo evil on me, or this tale of turd is *exactly* what he was referring to, but just couldn't bring himself to say. How many people would be scared of getting themselves knocked up if they knew that, at some point, they would have to reach into their child's ass and pull a demon-poop out for them? Whether it be boogers, pus, vomit, or a turd the size of a Buick (I'm serious. We could have thrown it in the ocean, given it its own name, and claimed it was an island), it always lessens the blow to know that we do all of these disgusting, awful, and nightmarish things because these are our babies and we don't want to see them suffer. Because we are their parents, and like it or not, we love them, and it's our job.

There I sat on the couch, years after the poo smell had finally washed from Thomas's hands, the kids still screaming for no reason, and the truth became very clear. Not only were both of my jerkwad children going to get their asses stuck in time out, but I then realized that a little part of us died on that disgusting night. I'm not sure if that part was my sense of smell, my gag reflex, or my pride, but we were forever changed. Maybe it broke us; like a horse . . . or our poor secondhand couch back when I was pregnant. Never again would we be able to consider ourselves just Jenny and Thomas, rebel twenty-somethings—the retired musician and the database administrator. The moment Thomas and I resolved to pull poop out of this red-faced little humanoid creature that *we* had created together, we stopped feeling like we were playing house and started feeling like Holden's parents. Mommy and Daddy.

After a harrowing ordeal like that, we would never again be able to deny it in our own heads. Only a parent or a medical professional would do what we did . . . and maybe someone that had lost a bet, but that's it! Parenthood is understanding that to keep from *going* crazy, you have to accept that you already *are* crazy. And also understanding that you can say things like that, that make absolutely no sense, but make total sense at the same time.

For years, I'd joked about the brain-killing effect kids have on any person who has one, but could it be that mine was so far gone that I'd been owning the shit out of this (pun intended) "mom" thing all along and just not giving myself the credit or even realizing it thanks to mommy-brain in all of its forgetful and dopey glory? I'd been waiting for some "big change" to jump out and smack me in the face, but like the poop stuck up Holden's butt, something so big wasn't going to be quite that easy.

CHAPTER **21**

I SHARED MY UTERUS—ISN'T THAT ENOUGH?

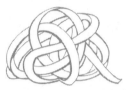

LOOKING BACK, THE WHOLE SMOOSHY-GUSHY lovey-dovey vomity *Brady Bunch*-ish "we are a loving, selfless family and so we share *everything*" bullshit that I worked so ridiculously hard to enforce in this house for the sake of my sanity may not have been all I originally thought it was cracked up to be. I was *wrong*?! How could it be?! My sharing free-for-all *does* have exceptions. Oh yes, it does. Like every law, there are loopholes. You just have to be sneaky enough to know where to look to find them.

I still insist that, *usually*, I have no problem sharing with the kids. Even things I love and don't have much of. Mi casa es su casa—and su came out of my vagina so I kind of have a soft spot for you. Those giant eyes with the ridiculously long lashes help, too. Really, I should be mad that little boys have longer eyelashes than me and never share a damn thing with them out of spite, but I do it out of love . . . and sometimes guilt. Okay, a *lot* of times guilt. Frequently, I found myself giving away nearly all of what I had just because I wanted to enjoy it in peace (read: so they would shut the hell up and stop bugging the crap out of me), and that is when I discovered the loophole. The glorious loophole—not to be confused with a Glory Hole. Don't you go confusing it with that!

Sure, children, I'll share everything with you! If you see me eating or drinking something, go ahead and ask for some! Sharing is awesome! If you *don't* see me eating something . . . boom! There it was. Shiny, and wonderful, and calling to me from afar. My new bestie: the loophole. What the kids don't *see* you eating, you don't have to share! They'll never even know!

It was ingenious! How could it *ever* fail? (Insert maniacal laugh here.)

I started out small, as not to alert the natives to my covert missions; short stop-offs in the pantry with the door open, blocking the children from seeing me as I ever-so-slowly reached my hand into a bag of potato chips, crammed them into my face, and speed-walked away before they would ever even *think* to ask what I was doing. Those damn kids, though. They are perceptive! It didn't take them long to catch on. Once they recognized the unmistakable sound of crinkling cellophane or plastic wrappers, sneaking around just out of plain sight wasn't gonna cut it anymore. Curse their sensitive virgin ears, free of the damage that shitty headphones and crappy rock concert speakers cause after years of exposure!

It was then time for Plan B—and I'm not referring to the over-the-counter shit you do the walk of shame to obtain after a drunken night of you know what. I'm talking about something far more serious: the fake out. I would buy them things they thought were super-special treats and make an enormous production over rewarding them with it. You and I both know that compared to the shit that *we* love, crap designed for little kids today tastes like fucking garbage. I don't care if it's healthy: if I want to snack on something (or my uterus is clawing my insides while screeching "salt!!"), I will not be satisfied with lightly flavored cardboard bullshit or sugar-free, low-fat, no-flavor, full of *lies* "candy" vomit. No. I want the *good* shit, and it is then that Suzy Shares-A-Lot suddenly takes a well-deserved vacation.

Lucky for me, the kids love that crap; they go insane for it—which gave me just enough of a window to hoard chocolatey goodness in my cheek like a chipmunk preparing for hibernation while those fart heads were distracted with their special "reward." By the time they looked to see what I was doing, they couldn't tell *what* was in my mouth and just assumed it was what they were having at the time. Stupid little kids! I win! Or . . . maybe I started celebrating too soon. Just like their ears, their noses are pretty fucking sensitive, too.

"Mommy, what's your breath smell like?"

These brats are like chocolate bloodhounds. You can't fool them! Sure, you can *try* to lie to them; tell them you are so naturally sweet that, without eating a thing, your breath smells of sugary deliciousness. You can even try to mask the stench of Cheetos by biting into an onion (No, I have not tried that. Seriously! I haven't!), but eventually, the ruse is up. No way is Mommy crunching on onions in the middle of the day unless she's an alcoholic or mega-preggo. Personally, I'd rather them find out that I was sneaking snacks than brewing a new ankle-biter in the depths of my belly. When none of the tricks I'd learned worked anymore, the spiral of shame began. . . . Only, I wasn't so ashamed. I know what you're thinking: Lady, you're already pretty low if you're seriously considering biting into onions simply because you don't want to share some fucking Cheetos, but lemme tell you, that ain't even close to the bottom here.

Everyone who knows me, even as only an acquaintance, knows that I am obsessed with the fall season, and it has nothing to do with how annoyed I get during the hot months at the epic amount of boob-sweat I produce when I don't even have any boobs. It doesn't even have anything to do with the weather; I *hate* fall weather. It can go fuck itself *and* the horse it rode in on. I have only one word for you that describes my love: pumpkin. For three months a year, I shove as much pumpkin into my face and down into my belly as the human body will allow. It's a wonder Gene Wilder's version of Willy Wonka doesn't show up and cart me back to his factory after mistaking me for a bright orange Oompa Loompa; I frickin' *love* pumpkin. It's an unhealthy one-sided love, and I don't even care. I will try just about anything pumpkin flavored (though I do *not* recommend pumpkin fudge. Barf.) or pumpkin shaped, and I've even been tempted to chomp on things that are pumpkin scented. The point of this story is not the pumpkin, but that I love it more than anything else, and as much as I love my spawn . . . if I find pumpkin deliciousness, it is *mine*. Screw you, Suzy Shares-A-Lot! You can't have any either!

Don't make a frowny disappointed face; it's only around for a limited time!

It had been well over a month since pumpkin season had ended when I was strolling through the grocery store and stopped at the super-clearance Christmas section (shit on sale is *always* awesome) when I spotted them: Pumpkin Pop Tarts. I'd been looking for those bitches for months and had begun to think they were nothing more than a myth. You better frickin' believe that I snatched up that box and did a Snoopy dance right there in the middle of the store. I imagine it resembled a really shitty touchdown dance. I once had rhythm, but months of pregnant waddling and two vaginal childbirths ruined that.

Those delicious morsels of pumpkinny Pop Tart were so good that I hoarded them, only breaking one out to eat every few weeks. Being the kind and generous mother that I am, I even shared a teensy bit of these rare commodities with the kids. Not the husband, though. One morning I caught him trying to sneak out the front door with a pack and let me just say—he should feel *so* lucky he handed them over to me without pulling back a bloody stump.

Everything was hunky-dory in shares-ville until there was just one pack left. Knowing this would be the last I'd get to taste them in all of their delicious glory for nearly another year, no one was to touch them. *No one.* I even pretended they didn't exist for a while, just so everyone would forget and I could have them all to myself without anyone bugging me. I'm not proud of what I did next, but sometimes a parent's gotta do what a parent's gotta do. I waited until both children were sufficiently cracked out on the TV, quietly crept into the pantry, grabbed the last remaining pack of my precious pumpkin Pop Tarts, and snuck into the bathroom.

There I sat; perched atop my porcelain throne, stuffing my face as quietly as I could and praying no one heard me. Eating in the same place I unleash my bowels might seem kind of low; mixing business with pleasure is often frowned upon, but you know what? I didn't even care; not one little bit. Why? Because that shit was all *mine* and I don't even allow that word in my house! As I inhaled the last morsel, giggling to myself upon realizing I had actually been victorious, it all fell into place. Who the hell in their right mind does this kind of wacky-ass thing? Who would ever even *think* to do this, and giggling crazily to themselves while they did? A nearly-insane sneaky ass *parent*, that's who. A mom. Me! Curse that loud ass cellophane wrapper! Before I could finish relishing my new-found appreciation for the title I'd avoided wearing for so long, before I could even finish choking down the final tart, I heard an enemy approaching.

"What you doing in there?"

Crunch, crunch, munch, gulp.

" . . . Pooping . . ."

My children now think I have bowel issues and crunchy turds, but y'know what? It was completely, totally, 5,000 percent worth it! I have since improved upon my snack-sneaking techniques, and no longer do I eat where I shit, but there may be a desperate time that times calls for desperate measures, and I will not hesitate to climb atop the toilet again. There are some cookies I just refuse to share. Hello, Girl Scouts? I'd like to request a secret delivery!

Stuffing my face on the crapper opened my eyes. That may be the weirdest sentence I have ever typed, but it's true! Why is it that we always have the most honest and true realizations, and make all of life's important decisions, while in the bathroom? Out with the old, in with the new? This was the first real time I'd done something that screams "mom" . . . and I wasn't embarrassed about it. There was no real shame-spiral, or self-loathing, or staring my old tired-ass face in the mirror and wondering what had become of me. Actually, it was . . . awesome. Seriously awesome.

The hoarding, the sharing (and *not* sharing), the scheming, the poop extracting, the grocery store vacationing, the tricking, the crying at the dumbest shit ever-ing. These are all things I've had recurring nightmares about. Okay, not really, but it's exactly who I swore I didn't want to be. At that moment, I didn't really see what was so wrong with it anymore. Are pumpkin Pop-Tarts that life-altering? As much as I love them, I don't think that's what was going on here.

If all of that wasn't proof enough, I *definitely* knew my life had forever been changed (more so than the actual act of giving birth to life) when a fellow mom or dad would say *"secret cookies"* and I was instantly aware that they weren't referring to flavored lube or some kind of foreplay. Let's face it—foreplay these days, for the ragged haggard parent, usually consists of brushing your teeth and half-conscious dry-humping. When I ask my husband to double-stuff me, it means I'm asking him to get his ass out of bed and go grab that pack of Oreos in the sock drawer.

CHAPTER 22

THE MANY MYSTICAL USES OF MOM SPIT

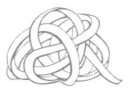

MAYBE I DIDN'T GET THE little girl I had always dreamed of, but I guess *someone* was listening when I said I wanted my children to take after me because my kids, bless their little hearts, are downright foul. They burp, they fart, and it doesn't matter where we are or who is listening, they feel the need to announce it. And never with that inside voice I've tried so hard to teach them. Those grody little children (and I use that term loosely some days) eat hair, boogers, toenails, and ancient Skittles they find on the floor of public places. I have still not gotten over the time my sweet baby found a dead bug in our living room and shoved that sucker directly into his mouth and I had to go diving in to retrieve it. They are disgusting-childhood-me to the eleventh power. Point? Be careful what you wish for!

While some people, my younger self included, may fool themselves into thinking that having girls means no farting at the dinner table, the truth is that kids are *all* nasty regardless of gender. Just ask me; I'm the little girl who spent most dinner times in the bathroom because I belched in the middle of the main course and was sent away until I could act like a lady. Most times I didn't return.

If I didn't know better, I would be convinced that when kids touch certain things, like dirt or mud or any kind of food, it changes the object's chemical compound. Instantly it becomes a cement-like substance that is seemingly *impossible* to remove. The shit simply will *not* come off, and it becomes absolutely indestructible. At first, you yank out a baby wipe, because you never leave the house without them, and over time you have become acutely aware that baby wipes are frickin' fantastic. They can take stains out of jeans! Sticky fingerprints off walls! Bring about world peace! Fine, maybe they aren't *that* powerful, but I wouldn't at all be surprised if they could polish up tarnished old silver . . . but who even uses that shit anymore? A more relevant use today is *obviously* baby asses and faces. Duh.

Once children are older and crapping in toilets instead of freshly changed diapers (or so you hope), the necessity to carry a ginormous baby bag with a bunch of junk you'll never use—but will bring just in case because you feel all panicky and paranoid about what *could* happen but is highly unlikely to if you don't—lessens greatly. I am to the point now where I just shove random junk in my purse, say "screw it!" to the rest, and run out the door. If shit is gonna happen, it's gonna happen (pun most definitely intended); I'll find a way to manage without the twenty-five-pound baby bag. I am *Mom* after all, right? We make it work!

The "Screw It!" philosophy has turned my purse into a science experiment. After a few months, I may find a half-eaten lollipop, a pack of smashed up saltines, a couple of curiously hairy Goldfish crackers, and a plastic banana at the bottom of my purse and have no idea when or how they even got there in the first place. I'm pretty sure if you dig deep enough, you'll find Jimmy Hoffa's body, but never have I found old, dried-out wipes that died a slow death in the bottomless pit that is my purse; I can't even remember the last time I used one. As weird as it sounds, the end of wipes makes me sad. I have given up on my babies being babies! I need them back! But not for sentimental reasons.

I *should* have wipes at all times because, without them, what am I left with when one of my precious boys gets their face caked in whatever they can manage to find on the floor, or by digging around in my purse because they think everything of mine is up for grabs and therefore becomes fair game to klepto? I could cart them off to the bathroom, but we've already extensively covered just how much that is not going to happen; it's a lot of frickin' work, and for very little payoff. Once they're in there, they'll insist on having to use it, and what was *intended* to be a two-minute ordeal turns into fifteen, and that's just unacceptable. Mama has clearance racks to raid! Maybe if you're lucky there will be a water fountain close by, but much like hair ties and bobby pins, you can never find those damn things when you really need them!

There is truly only one option left: the dreaded act of licking your very own thumb and rubbing that shmutz away.

Am I the only one who can't remember my high school teachers' names, but have vivid recollection of my toddlerhood? Somehow, I doubt it. Among those oddly prominent memories are *many* of my mother wiping various matter off my face with her thumb. As is the fact that she had *terrible* coffee breath, which I was delighted to tell her about any time she came within sniffing distance. Coupled with this is the absolute disgust I felt any time I saw that thumb invading my airspace. Due to this disgust and *repeated* offenses by my Mom, no matter how many times air traffic control told her to turn her ass around because she was absolutely, positively *not* cleared for landing, to this very day, I have and will always hate the smell of spit. Yes, the smell.

Not that I know anyone who *likes* it . . . or will admit to liking it, at least . . . but I *really* hate it. Even in my "I'm dumb, young, and slutty—let me make out with everything!"

phase, I'd have to tell those overly horny dudes to quit because I simply couldn't take the smell any longer. I liked to blame that on having "high morals," though. Whatever helps you sleep at night!

Years of my childhood were spent tormented with the thumb of doom. I spent years wondering to myself, *Why?? Why is this terrible woman doing this to me? What did I ever do to deserve her spitting on my face? She doesn't love me anymore! Can't she just use water? She's trying to kill me!* You can imagine the horror I felt when any dude came at me with his tongue out like he was going to wash my face rather than kiss it. (I just grossed myself out.)

At that moment, I made a promise to myself and to my future children. The one promise we parents should *never* make because it always comes back to haunt us; my famous last words:

I will never do this to my children!

Those words must taste like ten slices of calorie-free cheesecake because I am constantly eating them, and I tell myself they are delicious, but they're full of lies!

With all that said, even when I sat back and really thought about it, I could still never quite comprehend what the deal was with spit from a parent's mouth. Did it have some kind of unknown combination of periodic elements that could take paint off of a wall, but just hadn't been patented by a billionaire mogul yet? Is that why *every* mother, father, and grandmother seems to use it? What's so hard about walking to the nearest water source, wetting a napkin, and wiping dirt off a face that way? What on *Earth* could possess a grown ass adult to be so nasty as to spread their fucking *spit* all over their kids' faces? This made no logical sense to me.

It wasn't until the day I was out with my kids in tow (when are they not?), happily minding my own business (because for once they weren't being total shitbricks in public), when I noticed there was something on one of their face's that did not belong there; something crusty in appearance, but indistinguishable. If I had to give it an educated guess, it was probably a mixture of soil, snot, day-old milk, and a touch of evil. Yes, kids are *always* filthy little things, but that day in particular, the crust bugged me. Like it was staring into my soul . . . taunting me. Laughing at me because I no longer carried wipes in my purse and a water fountain or bathroom was nowhere in sight, but there *were* a ton of strangers around and I had the crusty kid. Oh *hell* no. You will not beat me today, indistinguishable mega-crust! I will not have the gross, crusty kid!

If I am ever questioned under oath about this incident, I will swear that what happened next was completely involuntary; I was possessed by the spirit of picky grandma's past! They're so judgy and mean! They *made* me do it! I am not my mother!!

Without even thinking, as though it were totally natural to me, as though I'd done it a million times before, I licked the pad of my thumb, put it to his cute, yet puke-worthy dirty face, and wiped that crust away. I felt something; it wasn't guilt, or shame, or wanting to shake my fist at my mother for getting into my head . . . It was a magic. In an instant, spit made total sense to me. What once was a long and tedious obstacle with flaming hoops and spiked hurdles to get through had just been reduced to a three-second lick of the thumb and graze across the face. Let us just forget that now the indistinguishable crust was on my finger. Some things are better left unsaid.

Mystified, I had to wonder if my spit had the power of a jackhammer, to so quickly and efficiently remove cement from the corner of a child's mouth—something I had to scrub the fuck out of to get off with anything else. Just as quickly as I'd wiped that gunk away, I decided it was best not to ask silly questions about something so wonderful and powerful. Did I forget to mention that it's *free*? You can't forget free. Baby wipes might be awesome, but something to wipe crap from tiny butts and crust from tiny faces should not cost what I'd expect to pay to wipe an elephant's ass.

While maybe I should have been feeling remorseful for putting my poor child through the same thing my mom tortured me with when I was little, something I had sworn never ever *ever* to do. . . . It was just too easy. Did I mention easy? Why would I go out of my way to run to the bathroom for some stupid face crust when I have an endless source of cleansing liquid right in the comfort of my own mouth? Spit doesn't take up *any* room in my purse. My poor old back thanks me tremendously.

Sure, my kid might reek of saliva for the remainder of the day, but it's *fast*, and in parent-world, fast is worth its weight in gold. It's also worth a little bit of childhood humiliation like the kind I experienced so long ago. Like it or not, kiddos, you're gonna have to deal with me smearing my spit on your face from now until well after it begins to embarrass your asses in public. Not just because it works, but for payback purposes for all the times you spit up directly onto my face (although it *is* a nice fringe benefit). Just be thankful that, on occasion, I ask "yours or mine?" Even though your spit fails miserably, at least I give it a fighting chance! You're welcome.

Now, as far as any real magical properties that parental-spit may have to it? I cannot confirm nor deny this, even though it does remove things that professional-grade crap claims to be able to, yet doesn't even come close to the raw, natural power of parental saliva. While testing my patience one day, my wonderful oldest child—who definitely knows better—decided to decorate my floor with marker. Yes, the markers that were off limits. I told Holden to lick his boogery little finger and rub that mess off of my nice, previously clean linoleum. He looked at me like I'd been snorting Lysol, but gave it a whirl, probably out of sheer curiosity. At the time, we were still in the "Mommy knows best" stage, or as I like to call them, the good ol' days. It didn't work, and in typical bratty fashion, he decided whining about it was the best course of action to take instead of oh, y'know, trying again? How absurd! Unthinkable!

I sauntered over, confidently licked my finger in stereotypical Mommy-fashion, and the marker came right off.

Gone! Poof! Presto! Bow down to me, my faithful crotch-blossoms!

Ahem. You go ahead and judge for yourselves on that last part there, but I, for one, am a believer. A new low? I think not. Fast and free; you simply can't argue with that. Had I not been so preoccupied with my sweet, spitty victory, I would have noticed that I'd just fallen headfirst down the rabbit hole and there would be no saving me. I would never be heard from again! This was the end of me as I knew it! The *horror*! Okay, okay, I'm being dramatic. Would you expect any less? In reality, I was finding my way *out* of the rabbit hole I'd dug for my stupid self. Because I was stubborn. And wrong. Yeah, I said it! See? Not all women refuse to admit when they're wrong. Just don't go expecting this shit on a regular basis.

CHAPTER 23

OH MY GOD, I AM MY PARENTS!

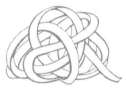

WHEN I WAS TWENTY-ONE, I got my very first pair of glasses. I'd been noticing that my vision wasn't quite as clear as I thought it should be, but I had no idea just how blurry I was seeing the world until I slid them on for the first time. The only time I ever experienced something like this again was when I could finally admit to myself that I'd had my head up my ass for years. The change I'd been waiting for so long to occur so that calling myself a "mom" wouldn't give me a full-body shudder? There was nothing to wait for; it had already happened. Duh! How the hell else would I have been able to do all of the nutty, revolting, and impressively inventive things to make it this far without snapping?

I was doing these weird, and possibly even demented, things and feeling mortified but laughing at the same time. The hell? It was all there, right in front of me, and I couldn't see it because I thought I had to fit into some stupid ass mold while shaking pom-poms to wear the "mom" crown. The mold I thought my mom fit into all this time didn't even frickin' exist! I certainly never got a citation that said, "Nope. Can't call yourself Mom until you get the minivan!" If I was wrong about there being a mold all this time, chances were that I was wrong about my mom all along, too. This also may have meant that I wasn't some "rebel" like I thought I was, bucking against the parenting stereotypes. Maybe I'd just been slowly forming my own non-moldy mold, just like my own mom? Crap.

I'm going to go ahead and assume my experience growing up was nothing other than ordinary. I have one older brother who was a total asshole to me and the standard hideous family minivan (dubbed The Silver Slug). I had parents who seemed to love each other one day and want to punch each other in the junk the next, a cat and a dog that fought like cats and dogs . . . and then there was my mom, who I swore was absolutely humiliating.

In typical tween (which there weren't fancy nicknames for, and we were all just "spoiled rotten brats") fashion, everything about my mom embarrassed me. Her giant permed hair with a back-teased tidal wave for bangs that was frosted within an inch of its life, the acid-washed jeans with ugly white tennis shoes and bunched down tube socks . . . everything. *She* thought she was fabulously stylish and prided herself on being good-looking, which she proved by telling a story about being pulled over by a police officer just to get her number. I don't exactly remember it that way, but any time I questioned it, she'd give me that look that said "say another word and I'll sell your bratty ass to the gypsies."

My mom was "awesome," but I didn't get it. I thought it was because I knew her behind closed doors, where you don't have to have things like patience, composure, or sanity understanding. I thought the world was full of stupid idiots for not seeing how evil my mom actually was. She was *ruining* my life. She was one step away from throwing me in a cold shower and beating me with a wire hanger; and for what?

So what if, at seven years old, I lined up the neighborhood kids into two groups and had one yell "Ass!" and the other yell "Hole!"—*I* didn't say it! Not innocent little me! Grounded. Ruining my life!

So what if, in first grade, I threw a wooden block up at a beehive in a tree while waiting for the bus, and some dumb turd walked under it as the block was coming back down and it bonked him on the head? I didn't throw it *at* him! Not my fault! Banned from the bus for a month *and* grounded. Life ruiner!

Who cares if I belch at the dinner table when no company is over? Who are we trying to impress here? Don't make me drink things that put bubbles in my stomach! Sent to time out in the bathroom while everyone else got dessert. Mom! Why are you trying to ruin my life??

Was it really so awful that I wrote about my "mean mommy" in my pink diary covered in illustrations of kittens? That was *private* and not intended for eyes other than my own! It's your own damn fault for invading my privacy. Life. Ruiner. Maybe *you* should be punished!

So I didn't tell you that I was going to the church's playground a mile down the road, and you didn't know where I was for hours. And? That playground was awesome and you wouldn't let me go to it because, according to you, it was "too far away." Well, maybe you shouldn't be so strict!

The worst, most heinous of offenses by my mother in my small child brain always occurred at meal time. She must have *only* done this because she wanted to punish me for yet another thing that was not my fault, but once a week, she would make meatloaf. I *hated* meatloaf. It tasted like barf. Not just any barf, mind you, but the dry chunky kind; the kind that has you spitting for an hour just to get it all out of your mouth. *Every week*. Why would this woman, giver of my life, make something she *knew* I hated so often if she loved me? And *trust* me—there is no way she did not know about this hatred. And then, on top of that, to put *lima beans* as the side dish??

No one likes lima beans!

Mother! Not Mommy, not Mom, but *Mother*—why are you trying to ruin my life?

To make matters worse, every time she would serve this horrid concoction, and every time I would tell her that there was no way on God's green earth I was going to eat it—that I would rather starve; I would rather die! Can't you just make something I *like*? I'm gonna tell on you. I don't know to *who*, but I *will!*—she would always respond with five words. Five words that, when put together, I grew to hate more than any other words in the entire English language:

"Like it or lump it."

It was a phrase I heard my grandma use from time to time, but never knew what it meant until used on me. It meant I was *not* going to get my way. You either eat what mommy made and like it—no complaining allowed—or you sit back like a lump on a log and get *nothing*. When faced with those two unattractive options, along with a growling stomach, I very rarely lumped it. I ate that gross, barfy meatloaf and those mealy, putrid limas (since back then we still believed in adhering to the rules of the "clean plate club" to either earn dessert or be able to leave the table), but I *didn't* like it. Devil woman.

When I had kids, I would *never* make them eat barfy meatloaf or putrid limas! I would *never* make them like it or fucking lump it! I would never be a mean ol' mommy and try to ruin their lives! Never ever!

I wrote that in my diary, too.

Grounded again.

Fast forward a gajillion years, and along came baby—*my* baby. Holden spoiled me. I didn't think he did, what with seven-hour marathon screaming fits nearly every night for the first six months, but apparently that earned me some kind of weird karma points because he was seriously one of the best toddlers ever. Terrible twos, my ass! He was calm, he went to sleep at night without a battle royale, he didn't have a bad attitude, and he was never a stingy brat when it came to other kids. Oh, and he would eat *anything*. He was my precious fat-roll-covered garbage disposal.

Even if you could tell by the look on his squishy little face that he thought whatever he was eating was the most awful thing he'd ever tasted, he would still devour it while telling you it was yummy. Most days I was convinced he was defective; he was just *too* good to be normal. And I was right, because that biatch karma, who seems to take forever paying visits to those who actually deserve it, swooped back down and decided to make up for her oversight by plaguing my second child.

Parker is the single most frustrating creature I have ever encountered. He is the cutest, most loving little human, too, which is lucky for him because when it comes to food, he turns into a monster. Like a gremlin after you get it wet or feed it after midnight, he transforms into a beast right in front of your eyes. This isn't to say it's *all* his fault; Parker spent the majority of his infancy very ill, and due to that, developed an aversion to food. After more than a year of occupational and speech therapy, at his very last appointment, we were given the all-clear and told that any remaining reluctance or refusal to eat (though he had progressed amazingly) was due to age and stubbornness. Basically, the dreaded and much-feared terrible twos had finally reared its ugly head. Our kid was a certified asshole. His therapist didn't exactly use those words, but that's definitely what she meant. I just know it.

The *actual* words she spoke? I was now the proud, yet frustrated mother of a picky eater. I still like mine better.

Each night, we would gather around the dinner table, Thomas tired from work, and me, tired from two bull-headed children, and try to have a peaceful meal, only it was *never* peaceful. It was a battle of epic proportions. You'd expect Parker to sit there and refuse veggies like any other child, but the kid *loved* veggies! It was absolutely every single other edible thing on the face of the earth that was the problem. He liked cheese, but not melted cheese. He liked bacon, but only in gross imitation bacon bit form. Picky McPickerson requested noodles at every single meal, but if you dared to put *any* kind of sauce on them and then dangle a forkful of it near his mouth, you'd be met with a shaking red howling baby head. If you were *really* unlucky, you'd be wearing it. Noodle-boob is not a new fashion trend.

I won't lie here and claim to have patience by the buttload, but when it came to Parker and food, it's something you *had* to have an abundance of. That, and super manipulation skills. Basically, I had to be a car salesman—only when I bribed the little haggler, I actually made good on my promises. Once we got that all-clear from his therapist, though, that Supermom patience naturally began to wear thin a hell of a lot faster. Too many times to count, I have had conversations that ended with "but you *loved* this yesterday!" As dinner crept dangerously close to the hour mark when Thomas, Holden, and myself had finished fifty minutes prior, that patience thing became even thinner than my thighs before popping that kid out.

The moment I let go of "patient Mommy" and made way for "frustrated bordering on snapping mean Mommy" (which I will admit that, at times, I enjoy) was also the moment when I could no longer sit at the table quietly until this kid eats his second fucking bite of *one* chicken nugget. Would Parker one day angrily write about this in his diary? Mean Mommy is for your own good, kid! Seriously—it does *not* take that long to chew one bite! What are you doing in there? Trying to see if you can liquefy poultry? Do you want a nugget milkshake? That's fucking nasty! Just swallow it so we can be done already! For the love of shit!

"But I don't want any more! I no like it!"

"You can like it or *lump* it!"

I swear to the stars in the sky, the world stopped spinning and those five words tumbled out of my mouth like I'd said them a thousand times before and echoed around the kitchen like I'd just yelled them into the Grand Canyon. A look of puzzlement spread over that stubborn and whiny, yet loveable, little face. He may not have had *any* idea what I was talking about, but he knew I meant business. We finished dinner in record time that night, and I knew then that the unthinkable had occurred.

I had opened my mouth and, instead of my own voice, my mother's had come out.

I felt a strange resolve within myself that night. Did I finally pass the test? Was this whole insane ordeal just a rite of passage to get it into my head that some things come naturally (as much as I *hate* it when people say that), and some are passed down from generation to generation because they *work*, but "Mom" was still whatever I wanted it to be? Had I finally been initiated into the secret parent club with the secret handshakes, secret phrases to get kids to obey, and the secret cookies?

Yes, the dark side really *does* have cookies. They are delicious *and* homemade.

CHAPTER **24**

A MOTHER'S CURSE: THIS AIN'T YOUR PERIOD, LADIES

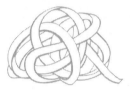

My PARENTS WERE CLEARLY PSYCHIC and could see my future
. . . or maybe they were witches and put a hex on me for
all the days and nights I, as they put it, "screamed like a
banshee" when I was a baby. Or, *maybe*, they used a time
machine they invented to travel through space and spy on
me so they'd constantly be able to say, with 100 percent
accuracy, "I told you so." because they already saw it happen. My mom easily could have been hiding a PhD under
those huge fucking bangs of hers. How else could they *possibly* predict absolutely everything that was ever going to
take place in my life as a parent?

There was one thing my mom, seer of futures, would say
to me nearly every time I found my ass in hot water with her
that never made a lot of sense to me while growing up:

"I hope you have a child *just* like you!"

Um . . . okay. That would be awesome, because I am
awesome and my kids won't hate me because I won't punish
them simply for their awesomeness. Who *wouldn't* want a
kid like me? What a silly thing to say! Am I supposed to be
scared or something?

I'm not denying that I have my moments of sheer idiocy.
Many of them, in fact, and this was definitely one. Cut
me some slack; I was young, innocent, and still believed

in Santa! Trust me when I tell you that if you laugh at a traditional parenting saying, it just multiplies the intensity for when the circle of life finally comes back around and it's your turn. No one ever warns us of that, though. If you ask me, this parenting business is all very hush-hush.

Kids always have this notion in their adorably devious little heads that their parents are the worst on the entire planet, and that one day, five million years in the future when they are finally as old as us and have their own kids, they are going to be the best parents *ever*. Not only are their kids going to be pictures of perfection (like them, *duh*), but they as adults will be loved by all children because there will be no bed times or curfew, ice cream for dinner, and chocolate chip pancakes every morning for breakfast. Screw fruits and veggies! I won't make my awesome "just like me" kid eat that nonsense! That's exactly what *I* thought way back when.

No, Mom and Dad. I won't understand when I get older, and you can't scare me! I will never join the dark side! Stupid, naive little me. If only I'd known about the cookies.

Somewhere after age twenty-one, common sense kicks in. Maybe it's a different age for everyone, but I have this sneaking suspicion it's when the majority of folks today turn the age they've been waiting for their whole lives—twenty-one! Legal! I can drink without getting in trouble! I'm an adult and I'm *free*! Once the shininess wears off and bills and responsibilities kick in, they realize this whole "adult" thing was not all it was cracked up to be, just like I did. It actually kinda blows in a lot of ways. And by a lot, I mean most.

We all break a little when we get paid and nearly every dime is already spoken for. No more going to the convenience store and blowing our allowances on Air Heads and Milky Ways, which causes you to begin longing for your childhood—the one you thought was so tough and unfair and was actually a piece of fucking cake. The store-bought kind, not the kind you have to make yourself. Basically what I'm saying is that it was *easy*. Why? Because we had parents who made it that way for us, and we never even noticed. We were too busy bitching about bed times and vegetables.

Wait just a damn minute! Does this mean my childhood was awesome, but *I* wasn't? That simply cannot be true! I was only sent to the principal's office a few times in my entire thirteen-year public school stint. I never got in trouble with the law, and my grades were always pretty good—that definitely means I was totally awesome and that a kid like me would be equally as such! I'm so dense sometimes.

From the age of eighteen on, I lived in my own place, paid my own bills, and considered myself to be pretty damn smart for being so self-sufficient at such a young age. I toured the east coast as a musician, moved to Los Angeles, and even found myself without a place to call home a few times. I'd been through a lot, but even with all those experiences under my belt, by the time I was twenty-two, nothing was more of a reality check than having a baby.

At first, every single thing on the face of the earth was a hazard. Once I got a decent hold of my overprotective nature (a.k.a. my crazy), I could see the beauty around me as my own child—the one *I* created and brought into this big scary world—and experienced it all for the first time. There's something magical about being able to see the world through a child's eyes. Childbirth, explosive diapers, months of little to no sleep . . . You're never really ready for the day that your precious, perfect baby, with their big bright eyes taking in all of their surroundings, and that sweet and innocent smile that you can't ever get enough of, pulls the rug out from under you.

This baby, at times, is so perfect that you aren't really sure where they got all the cute from because nothing has *ever* been so cute. Certainly this wasn't like when you were younger and your parents were always yelling at you that they hoped you had a kid "just like you," as if it would be a spawn from hell. This thing is way too cute to be a demon! You *must* have been right way back when you remarked how super awesome that would be. . . . And then, suddenly, precious, sweet, innocent, perfect little mini-you unleashes upon you a level of sass only matched by your very own childhood shitheadedness, and you quickly come to the realization that "I hope you have a kid just like you" was not something to look forward to. It was not a *blessing*. It was not *awesome*, and neither were you. It was a *curse*.

I may have been what most people would consider a good kid if you look at my youth as a whole, but when looking back on it with the eyes of a parent, I am able to see things much differently; I can see it the way my parents saw it. I'm not happy to admit that I was a total brat. An evil, foul-mouthed, mood-ruining little jerk. The shame! What I lacked in acting out at school, I more than made up for in back-sass and attitude.

The first time Holden ever whined "That's not fair!" and stomped down the hallway, slammed his bedroom door, and said loudly enough for me to hear "I'm never doing that *ever* again!" I had flashes of myself doing the same *exact* thing. I knew then that the curse had been activated. You know the saying *I'm rubber and you're glue, everything you say bounces off of me and sticks to you*? It's silly, immature even, but that is how life and Karma treats parenthood. However nasty, sassy, or smart-assy you are as a kid will come back to haunt you once you have one of your own, and there's not a damn thing you can do to stop it. It is a curse passed down from generation to generation that we don't learn about until it's far too late to turn back.

My kids are quick-witted, overly-sensitive brats, and I only have myself to blame. Even though I'd love to blame Thomas, and his mother would love nothing more than to claim every tiny random part of their personalities for herself, these boys are *all* me. Right down to tripping over absolutely nothing and having to do random gravity checks. Sorry, kids! It's the curse at work.

More often than I care to admit, I am caught off-guard by just how quickly they snap back at me with logic that I just can't argue against, a common complaint about my mouth as a child. One time in particular, Holden was writing something about Spiderman on a piece of paper. I, being the helpful parent I am, informed him that his *p* and *d* were both backward. The response I got nearly knocked me out of my seat. He stopped what he was doing, sighed deeply, and said in a very dry and not at *all* snotty tone "I *know*, Mommy. I can't exactly erase crayon."

Well, excuse the fuck outta me!

On the one hand, he was absolutely right and I was a little proud with how fast he called me on it—that was smart! On the other, Holy Backsass, Batman! Of all the traits I hoped to pass down, brat was *not* one of them. I feared for my future dealing with that mouth. I take solace in knowing that the ultimate revenge will come in the form of my future grandchildren. And no, I'm not going to warn my kids first. And there it is! Right there! The full circle will be complete! The best part? Whenever the curse rears its ugly head via childhood attitude then? I can give those suckers back! Not my problem anymore! Move out of the way, dingle-berries! Gramma's going to bingo night!

CHAPTER 25

EVERYTHING BUT THOSE HIDEOUS TUBE SOCKS

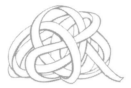

I NEVER THOUGHT IT WOULD happen; actually, I swore that it wouldn't. I didn't think that it *had* until I sat down however the hell long ago it was to start writing this book and it became a startling recurring theme: my parents really *were* right all along. Trust me when I tell you that not even I can believe I wrote that . . . and I'm not sure I'd ever admit it aloud or the gloating from my dad would be outrageously unbearable, but unfortunately, it is truer than true. All those times they told me that I'd understand when I was older why they did, said, and refused to let me do the things I wanted now made sense. The insane time-outs they swore were actually lenient but I likened to a lifetime jail sentence—shit, even how I feel about life, my youth, and my own kids—they pegged it all. All of it! If only they would have started an underground gambling ring out of it, they'd have both been millionaires by now.

If my mom were here today, she'd be having uncontrollable gigglefits as I proved her right every single day and the phone calls from me started pouring in cursing her for it. She'd be doing a gloriously extravagant victory dance. Even if she was sometimes harsh, it wasn't totally her fault. I maaaaaaybe *sorta*-kinda deserved it. My nickname for her back when I was an a-holey brat (much like mine are

137

now; coincidence?) was Bubble Butt. . . . Oh, and Beluga Whale once the summer months rolled around. It's no wonder the woman tortured me with embarrassment; I'd have done the same damn thing! In fact, I *do* the same damn thing now! I imagine myself in the future as a grandmother feeling completely vindicated in all the shit my kids are giving me grief about right now as it is happening to them. History *does* tend to repeat itself. At least I have that little notion to comfort me.

Parenthood is not an eighteen-year commitment; it is signing away the entire rest of your life. From the moment you conceive until your very last breath, you will be a worrying parent. Possibly even after. Who *doesn't* want to haunt the shit out of their kids? Whether it be your children or your children's children—it never ends! So much for the notion that once the kids move out on their own (if they ever do!), you're "done"!

Never before has my nose been rubbed in my eternal wrongness so hard as when it comes to toys. Now, I never saw my mom go totally spaz-crazy and tear the batteries out of a toy like it was the heart of her prey—and yes, I have absolutely done that—but she didn't seem to develop the same kind of seething hatred that I have for some of the ones my kids have. Maybe she was just better at hiding it, or maybe I was just too caught up in being a selfish worry-free little kid to even notice. It's even possible that I was trapped in that hideous whale dress she insisted I wear that I swore would be the death of me, screaming at the top of my lungs with no regard to the world, toys, or my mom.

My entire life, toys were simply things to play with. Nothing more. This playing included smashing them together, throwing them, sitting on them, crushing them, grinding them into dirt, riding on them when they were not at *all* built to be ridden, dunking them in water when they were not waterproof, and trying to make every last one of them fly—wings or no wings. Isn't that what they were for? Playing? *Playing* is a vast and broad term—or I thought so, anyway. Apparently I was dead-ass wrong. I played with my toys exactly how I saw fit, but somehow I always got in trouble for doing these things. What? Why? What did I do wrong? It's a *toy*! It's *meant* to be played with! You're crazy, lady! You are a *mean* ol' mommy! Man, that sounds so damn familiar, doesn't it?

Life loves to play cruel jokes on us, and just like my mean ol' mommy warned me that I'd understand when I had little punks of my own, and I thought she was totally full of crap because it was *soooo* obvious that she was just trying to get her way for no reason other than to protect her perfect record of being right—and also to be mean because she loved that shit—I finally got it. I hadn't wanted to, but that didn't make it any less true. That thick skull I was always told I had, that no amount of logic could penetrate, finally softened up and gave reality a chance to swoop in and punch me in the tit. I hear this happens to other parents once they pull their heads out of their asses, too, but at the time I was feeling pretty naked and alone once my security blanket of childhood obliviousness was ripped away.

Yep, a punch to the tit, alright. Reality sucker-punched 'em good and hard. Come to think of it, it may have been more like smashed. Smashed tits—not exactly the visual I was going for, but let's run with it, shall we?

Smashing—like what I find myself constantly walking in on for as long as my mommy mind can recall—with Parker taking one toy and beating the ever-living fuck out of another. He's just a kid, and a boy at that! They're *supposed* to do these kinds of destructive things. Totally normal . . . isn't it? Yeah . . . not so much. Instead of seeing a normal, innocent little boy banging around toys in a way that comes naturally to him and most other kids, I see money being sucked right out of his bedroom window.

What the hell? What are you doing? That is *expensive*! You stop that right now before you break it!

Oh! Hi, Mom! I didn't see you there in my subconscious. How long have you been there? What's that you said, my whole life? Okay then. Oh yeah, sure, make yourself at home! Have a fucking cookie while you're at it.

It's no wonder my mom's head nearly spun 360 degrees when she walked into the living room and caught me chopping off the heads of all of my Barbies with a piece of wood. It didn't matter that the heads easily pop on and off to begin with; it was that I was bludgeoning things she had spent money on, and money isn't something most of us enjoy carelessly tossing away. The value of the things I was beating to a pulp never even registered in my mind, just like it doesn't register in *my* kids' minds.

Since I lost my mom at nineteen, there wasn't really a time where she sat me down and imparted her vast knowledge and wisdom when it came to all-things parenthood to me. Other than repeatedly cursing me with evil spawn, we never talked about her eventual grandchildren or what to expect at all. Lucky for me, contrary to what my mom thought, I actually *did* listen to the things she said every now and then, so I picked up things here and there. *This* was the first time I ever unquestionably thought to myself, "Huh; maybe she *was* right," without wanting to slap myself afterward, that is. Mom was right. It felt good to say. It felt right.

I always thought if I ignored the feeling long enough it would go away—like a big red pimple—but that's not how life works. We get too tempted to pop those nasty things! That's when all the truth comes pouring out. (Okay, barf. Why did I write that?) A part of me is grateful that I finally understand my parents. I know now that they didn't always discipline me just because they *wanted* to. Disciplining kids sucks ass! Most of the time we parents wish we didn't have to at all; being the "bad cop" is exhausting. I know now that my parents disciplined me because they loved me enough not to want me to grow up to be a steaming sack of poop of a human being. That requires tough love at times—like when I, and now *my* little ones, bash expensive toys into oblivion . . . or drag around the family pet by the tail.

I *finally* understand that neither she nor my dad were just trying to pee on my good times to be mean, or because they hated things like fun and joy. (To me, my mom was evil, remember?) No, that's not the case at all. Now, I'm constantly trying to get that into my *own* kids' heads. The other part of me misses the me that had no concept of money, bills, or the dollar amount of a toy getting smashed to pieces in a fit of toddler glee. There's also this *itty-bitty* part of me that still hates being wrong and is still thoroughly weirded out every time I do something my mom would have done.

After all the fighting, denial, and flat-out refusal to accept my new reality, I could finally stand back, look at my life, and admit that my parents were right all along. Maybe not about *everything*—I mean, the woman wore *tube socks*—but a lot of other things they were spot on about. It was either that, or admit that I'd finally made good on all my threats and promises and had lost my damn mind. I think I picked the lesser of two evils here . . . most of the time. I just hope my kids realize this before I did, because otherwise, I am *so* screwed.

It's really too bad my mom isn't here to rub more of her rightness in my face like I know she would *love* to do . . . and to babysit the hellspawn she cursed me with!

CHAPTER 26

UNLESS YOU ARE DYING, DO NOT BLEED ON MY CARPET

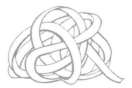

IF I COULD, I WOULD move back into my childhood home. It was spacious, in a nice neighborhood, had a pool, and was on a frickin' lake. Does it get much better than that? I loved everything about that house except for the door that led from the den to the garage. It was heavy, wooden, and didn't take much force to sound like you were angrily slamming it, which led to being sent to my room a lot more than I deserved to be. I loved my room, but only when I wanted to be in it. That was only the beginning of my deep-seeded hatred for that door.

One day, as I attempted to go out into the garage, that door—that, may I remind you, took zero force to slam—swung shut *ON* my heel. I cringe to even recall the memory of collapsing to the floor, looking at my foot, and seeing that the sonova-bitch had taken my Achilles tendon with it. Over twenty years later, I still have a scar. Something so horrific had to have my mommy running to my rescue, right? Oh, she ran alright, but only to protect her precious carpet from the blood pouring out of me. The age-old evil mom saying "Don't bleed on my carpet!" had reared its ugly head.

Look, y'all, it was *shag* carpet! Rusty, crusty orange shag carpet. My blood was probably an improvement!

Somehow, I managed to crawl off her precious carpet and swore to myself that I must have been adopted. My *real* mommy would be snuggling my tears away instead of lamenting over fifteen-year-old flooring. Without realizing it, I believe this experience colored my first few years of motherhood.

When Holden was born, I was what some people call . . . overprotective. Aw shit, let's just be real here—I was a full-on helicopter parent. Always watching, always hovering right above him, making sure nothing went wrong (because I was convinced something would the *moment* I took my eyes off of him). Once the kid became mobile, pretty much everything he did gave me a near heart attack. Multiple times per day I would find myself leaping toward him like an NFL pro to catch his bulbous dome, swearing he was *thisclose* to cracking it open. It's no wonder "new" moms look so frazzled all the time. Taking care of a little (and obnoxiously curious) one is manual labor and mental torture. It feels like you are constantly trying to diffuse a bomb that's set to go off any second. You don't know which second, but you *know* it's coming. And that it's probably full of poop.

Seasoned parents know that baby proofing only goes so far. You remove all sharp objects that could bonk poor baby's soft noggin, cover the outlets so baby doesn't electrocute him or herself, put *every* breakable object out of reach so there is absolutely no chance (or so you think) that baby will pull it down and be crawling over the shattered remnants. By the time you're done, your home has the appearance of a sterile mental ward. It feels like one, too.

For a while, it seemed like I would never get used to this drunken, uncoordinated zombie creature that came from my crotch like the chest-bursting beast in *Aliens*. My days were chockful of don't touches, look outs, no's, don't climb on thats, get away from theres, and more don't put that in your mouths than anyone other than a fellow helicopter mom could imagine. Exhausting doesn't even come close to describing the feeling. Nothing you do, short of placing lil' precious in a plastic bubble, wearing clothing made from Bubble Wrap, can keep them from getting hurt! They are *going* to fall, bonk their heads, and knock the wind out of themselves. (And you get the same feeling when they do this. Magic!) It sucks, but that is the reality of having kids.

Over time, you grow used to the bumps and thuds of these clumsy little b-holes, because they happen *so* often you begin to feel like you're training for a marathon—flying to their side to make sure they haven't broken a limb or an irreplaceable family heirloom. Through the racing heart, panting, and fatigue, another reality becomes clear: kids *bounce*.

That fact is proven to me pretty much every single day and almost always while I am busy doing something else, like working out. My kids must be trying to keep me from being the embarrassingly hot mom in the neighborhood. After working up a sweat one morning with my mockery of exercise, I dragged my nasty ass up the stairs so I could jump in the shower quick. I just needed to peel off the "I don't have boobs but they sure can sweat" clothes, and rinse off the funk I had acquired with a nice cold shower. I'm too lazy to wait for the water to get hot while I'm standing around naked and covered in non-boob sweat. I was standing in the bathroom naked with the bath water running, just about to climb in, when absolute mayhem erupted.

Not much earlier, I had asked Parker to come upstairs and get himself dressed while I got ready, but of course, he bitched and moaned about how he "wanted to *plaaaaaaaay*" and refused to follow me. I'd already learned the hard way to choose my battles wisely when it comes to mouthy, stubborn toddlers, so I didn't even bother trying to argue or push his bony ass up the stairs. It didn't take long after I'd stripped myself all the way down to my birthday suit to hear a loud *thump-thump-thump*. Since I'd left the bathroom door open (privacy is another battle not worth fighting), I craned my neck out and peered into the hallway and saw Parker and the dog making their way up the stairs. About damn time!

These things have the nasty habit of happening in the blink of an eye, so I truly have no fucking clue what went wrong once Parker got to the top of the stairs. All I know for certain is that he went flying into the door frame face first. If I were to make an educated guess, I suppose it could have been his enormous skull throwing him off-balance. Or maybe the dog, in a show of revenge for all the tail pulling and attempted horsey rides, cut him off and tripped him. Either one is highly possible because they both happen so frequently—but all I saw was a swoosh, a blur of blond hair, heard a cringe-worthy *bang*, and then there was a kid on the floor screaming bloody murder. These are the moments in parenthood that we cast all cares aside to get to our child's aid as fast as humanly possible. It doesn't matter what we're doing, how important, how far away . . . or even what we are, or are not, wearing.

There I am, butt-ass naked and totally disgusting—the water still running—leaping over to Parker to assess the damage. I would swear, with a smack like that, followed by the high decibel yelp he let out, that there was going to be blood. Lots and lots of blood; maybe even some missing teeth. The vision of my baby in public with a gapped grin and telling people he lost a fight with a bathroom door popped into my head. That sound could definitely have that ugly of a result, but if not that, definitely blood. I don't do well with blood; it makes me queasy.

I was totally prepared to do the typical little girl thing and shriek at the sight of an open wound and promptly faint. It's okay, I thought. I can do this! Just as long as he's alright, I can totally handle this. If I can survive childbirth, I can handle a little blood! High and low I searched for something, anything, to be wrong with him. He was telling me that his nose hurt, but it wasn't even red. The kid was completely unharmed. I may have *considered* the bubble-wrap helmet, but I didn't actually put him in one. How could this be? Thirty seconds later, he was trotting down the hallway with the dog, climbing onto my bed, and playing happily as though nothing ever happened. Still standing there, naked me was perplexed, but I shouldn't have been. This kind of crap isn't anything out of the ordinary. It isn't even the tiniest bit rare.

Even if there is blood, even if you could swear it was the most *awful* sound you have ever heard and it will haunt your dreams for eternity, give it a few minutes and everything will be back to normal. As normal as things can be with a crazy three-year-old, that is. Each and every time I find myself asking the same exact question: what the hell are kids made of?

It's eating away at me! I must know! I am 1,000 percent positive that if I took a flying face dive into a door frame, I would need an ambulance and reconstructive surgery. If I fell *half* of the amount of times with *half* the amount of force they do, I would not bounce. I would plop. Splat. Crunch. I would be in a full-body cast swearing to never leave the comfort of my bed again. The floor is made of fucking lava and I can't possibly get out! There would be no boo-hooing for two minutes and then joyously skipping off to play with toys, completely disregarding my busted lip, scraped knee, or a giant freakish lump on my head. There would be multiple broken bones, stitches, traction, and therapy—physical *and* mental.

Kids *bounce*! They are practically indestructible. Thousands of times, I have heard thuds coming from upstairs that are *so* loud it sounds like elephants bowling or a WWE cage match, and I've rushed to find my two sitting on the floor looking up at me with a puzzled expression because I am out of breath and frantic at the thought of them being hurt. Even if they are hollering like their asses have been lit on fire, it's typically because they're fighting over some stupid toy, not because they busted or broke something.

Slowly but surely, I built up a panic tolerance. It has served—not only my mental well-being—but slowed the progression of wrinkles on my face down to a crawl and stuffed the grays back into my scalp. Not stressed enough for that yet, body. Take it back! So what if I made that second part up? You get what I meant.

Twenty years ago, I didn't lose my foot in a freak door accident, but there's still something about heavy wooden doors that frighten me. Obviously I lived to tell the tale, so it couldn't have been *that* bad. Having to hire a professional cleaner to get my blood out of the carpet (even if it was *shag*, ugh) because I was screaming about how I was dying and wouldn't move? Yeah, I guess I can see why things played out how they did. Mom wins again. Skin grows back, booboos heal, bruises fade, and kids are crazy resilient. They are also horribly dramatic over the tiniest things. I would know.

I am a much calmer, more relaxed, and less spazzy mom now that I'm not always dashing to rescue someone who doesn't even need rescuing. At this point, I've been through so much that screaming no longer fazes me; I only get up for children at the sound of broken glass or the smell of smoke. Tough love, baby. Now get off my carpet before you bleed on it!

CHAPTER **27**

OF ALL THE THINGS I'VE LOST ... WAIT ... WHAT DID I LOSE AGAIN?

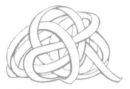

ONE OF THE EARLIEST THINGS I can remember is sitting on the kitchen floor of my beloved (if not slightly murderous) childhood home with my mom, who was holding up a spoon and a fork, encouraging me to repeat both words aloud. Much to her frustration, my "spoon" sounded more like "foon."

For the majority of my life, I thought that memory was from when I was four years old, but now that I have kids of my own who wouldn't shut the hell up at the age of two (even if it was 75 percent gibberish), I am aware this memory is likely from a younger age. This tells me one undeniable fact—I have an *amazing* memory! No, really! I do! I've never been good with names, but if I see your face *one* time, I can pick it out anywhere from that moment on. It makes for some awkward conversations when I tell someone that I have *absolutely* seen them before but can't remember their name. Stalker much?

Other than freaking the hell out of people, my memory is pretty damn awesome . . . or, I should say, was. It *was* pretty damn awesome, and then a child fell out of my vagina and my brain stopped functioning correctly. Ever since that day, I have felt not only my sanity, but the capacity at which my brains runs, slowly slipping farther and farther away. I don't know where my mind is going, but I'm pretty damn sure the kids took it.

Not long ago, I attributed this constant forgetfulness I've been experiencing to giving birth. I mean, you *are* pushing pretty hard—that has to account for a large loss of brain cells. I even liked to call it "post-preggo brain," but it's been years since the last time I bulldozed a baby out of my private parts; I can't place the blame there anymore. Those of us plagued with memory loss and extreme forgetfulness (and a vagina) refer to it as Mommy-Brain (or Daddy-Brain for those with wieners out there). Once Mommy-Brain takes complete hold of a person, they instantaneously become well aware of the ultimate level of duh they can, and *will*, reach. Living in denial about it takes far too much energy.

The loss of my once marvelous brain was the first life change, besides stupidly wider hips, that I acknowledged. This probably had less to do with accepting my mom-ness, and more with realizing that if having kids hadn't done this to me, I would have no one to blame my dumbness on, and thereby would just be dumb. That wasn't gonna fly!

It begins early—while we are expanding due to the growth of a baby in our belly. I like to believe that in order to develop their teeny brains, we had to sacrifice a little bit of ours. Okay, *okay*!! A *lot*! We mistakenly thought as soon as they tore through our nethers and re-lit the vacancy sign outside our uteri, that slowly, brain capacity would increase, and in turn, brain farts would fade away into the distance. Over time, we'd get back to our incredibly smart and charming selves (even if our hair was frazzled from repeated attempts to rip it out). And our wit! We'd be witty again!

Through talking to other parents over an extended period of time, we have all come to the shared conclusion that Mommy-Brain is a permanent condition. Try as you might to deny it, deep down you know the pause between clever retorts, forgetfulness, the filter we had to have to refrain from talking in disgusting detail about diarrhea, and "duh" moments are far more frequent than before. Those bitches have *not* reduced in the slightest as the years pass. I'm going to be dumb for the rest of my life! And I thought the stretchmarks were bad!

One year after the birth of my youngest crotchfruit, I was looking for a lighter so I could fire up a candle. Two little boys can create quite the putrid funk—one the average human would be desperate to get rid of. It was nowhere to be found. The first thought that popped into my head was that the husband unit took it. He's *always* taking it, so he must have it! I swear to the sweet baby Jesus that he took it and I am going to hurt that man! Any angrier and I would have turned green and Hulk smashed the shit out of the coffee table.

Thanks to that turdbreath, now I would have to smell funk all damn day long, and by the end of the day, I would be immune to it only because now *I* smelled like it. Gross! Four hours later, after endless streams of curse words that would make a drunken pirate blush, I found it. In my pocket.

Two years after my last stint in labor and delivery, I totally spaced on wrapping the "big" birthday gift for the boys. (They are two years and two weeks apart. Do you really think I'm gonna throw two separate parties when those kids don't even have their own friends yet? Oh hell no.) The one I'd spent months thinking about and tracking down. I was *so* excited to watch them open it so that I could see their eyes light up because they'd begged for this thing for months, and because I wanted one moment of "I am awesome!"-ness. I wanted my "#1 Mom" merit badge, damnit!

We got to the end of unwrapping the ridiculous amount of gifts they'd received when I realized I hadn't seen them open the grand finale gift. I panicked, thinking I'd left it at the toy store or maybe I never even got it out of hiding. With the way my brain was going, one is not wrong to assume the worst. Thirty minutes passed and I found the big mamma jamma gift tossed carelessly into the giant pile of crap they'd received that day, already out of its packaging. Since it hadn't been wrapped, the two little girls who were helping to open all of the boxes, and then removing all those infuriating twisty-ties, thought it had been opened already. I picked it up and showed it to Holden only to have him shrug his shoulders like it was no big deal. No lit up eyes, no big surprise, just a big fat *fail*.

Three years after the most recent vag-splosion and I'm afraid that my brain had only gotten worse. Having two kids that can talk, which means they can also argue until they're blue in the face, has a lot to do with the rapid deterioration of my mind. And also my patience. From that point through present day, I have done a large disservice to women by forgetting not only my wedding anniversary, but also how long Thomas and I have even been married. *He* had to correct *me*. How often does *that* happen? And how are we supposed to bitch at men about not making dinner reservations or bringing home flowers if Mommy-Brain has taken over and *we* are the ones always forgetting? In the pregnancy days (or as I like to call them, the dark ages), people told me this condition would get better over time. People are filthy fucking liars.

I can't even calculate the number of times I've had moments of "Where the hell is my—oh, there it is." Even more frequently than that, I have walked into a room to get something only to immediately forget what it was. If I'm *really* lucky, I'll remember what it was before I leave the room, but most days? Nothing. Memory is completely blank. You might think forgetting my wedding anniversary is the worst thing I could have done to my husband in this stage of deteriorating Mommy-Brain, but you'd be wrong.

We had lived in our current home for nearly two years and were still making empty promises to go to the hardware store to make an extra key. Upon moving in, we were only given one set of keys—for two people! Makes total sense. One key *obviously* went to the front door, but the other we still haven't figured the hell out. It could potentially unlock the doorway to Narnia for all we know. All I *do* know is that it doesn't unlock anything in this house. A second key to the front door would have been far more useful, if you ask me, but what do I know? I just live here.

Empty promise going unfulfilled, that one key went to me. It's not like I ever leave the house, and on the weekends we go out together, so it's no biggie for me to carry around the only key! Am I right, or am I right? Giving the one and only key to our front door to the most forgetful family member? I can't foresee anything bad happening! No way!

I remember one day when I was about four seconds from burning the house down, and desperately needed to get out of there. Our AC had gone out and it was nearing epic-buttsweat level hot in that place. To put it simply—I couldn't take it anymore! The house was a menopause simulator and if we didn't leave, I would end up spontaneously combusting. A genius idea popped into my boiling brain: we'll go out to dinner! What a perfect plan! I didn't have to cook, and it would keep us out of Buttsweat City for a pretty good chunk of time since Parker is the slowest eater on the planet. This is the only time his annoyingly slow eating habit has benefited us. I will *never* tell him that, but I'll take it!

The moment we walked out of the house and closed the front door, I knew something was wrong. I dug down into my purse for a moment and then had to deliver the bad news—my keys were still inside. This included the *only* key to the front door. Oops! How can I be expected to remember the keys all the time if I'm never the one driving? A little reminder would be nice!

Poor Thomas. He had to go into the backyard, get the ladder off the shed, climb onto the roof, and crawl through the upstairs bathroom window to get in. How did he know that would actually get him into the house? Well, let's just say that it wasn't the first (or fifth) time he's had to do it. And almost *always* right after it's rained. I swear the neighbors think I'm trying to kill the man, but I'm not! I promise!

Blame my uterus. That bitch is still pissed about having to grow a baby two times in two years, and ohhhhh *man* is her monthly revenge ugly. The penis at fault in this situation is *not* safe.

Don't count on a parent to remember what day of the week it is, what their own kids' names are at all times, or even how old they are. We are running on months to years of very little sleep. Even though the kids are out of us (physically, at least), I'm convinced there's an invisible umbilical cord attached to us, leeching off our energy. It's a pretty convincing indication that the brain after childbirth is permanently affected when I can remember exactly how many seconds it takes to perfectly warm up a baby bottle when I haven't had a baby in years, but have no idea what I had for dinner last night.

I've begun to wonder (as much as I can without straining myself) if I'll know when I slip from Mommy-Brain into age-related dementia with a heaping side of Alzheimer's. With the way things are going, it will likely be a smooth and completely unnoticeable transition. People say that obnoxious yellow animated square bastard lovingly referred to as Spongebob rots kids' brains, but kids rot *our* brains. That's my story and I'm sticking to it . . . until I forget that I wrote this, that is.

CHAPTER **28**

Making my kids need therapy, one day at a time

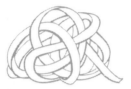

FOR YEARS, I LAMENTED THE fact that I didn't have my mom around for advice, to meet her grandchildren, or even just to call when nothing was going right and I just wanted my mommy. I still think it seriously sucks, and it probably always will; she would have made the most *hilariously* obnoxious mother-in-law, and the kind of smothering Grandma that I'd have to yell at to back the hell off. I'm not as sad as I used to be, though, because now I know she's always with me—and in a *perfectly* torturous way. She is my subconscious, always in my head, influencing the crap that comes out of my mouth. Or maybe she's the devil on my shoulder telling me to do evil mommy things . . . *deliciously* evil mommy things.

Parental enjoyment outside of baby's first words and other aww-worthy milestones tend to be few and far between. This is not to say that children are life-ruiners, but for a while, it might seem like they are the only entertainment you get, and they spend a hell of a lot of that time perfecting the art of the most obnoxious whine known to man. They don't call them the Terrible Twos, Terrorist Threes, and Holy *Fuck* Fours (and so on) for nothing. There comes a time in which a parent might have to be crafty when it comes to personal amusement. And I'm not talking the dirty kind here, people.

Thank you, evil mom on the shoulder; you are a true inspiration.

It would probably make me a horrible, terrible, and craptacular piece of work to claim that parenting is such an immensely frustrating and misery-filled job that we parents have to always take solace in the little things, for we have nothing else to brighten our days. It would also make me a liar because that is simply not true. Well, most of the time. I found that some days, it was just harder to find the bright spot than others—but—it can be done!

Those of us mere mortals who lack the patience of a saint, or the ability to turn off our ears amidst eardrum-shattering chaos, know that there will be days where we are literally counting the minutes until baby bedtime. During those horrible, terrible, sanity-shattering days is when we learn that while these little things are definitely not the *only* things we have to brighten our days, they are still far more awesome than we give them credit for. I may never have figured out what every baby cry meant, or why the hell their poop is full of seeds, but it didn't take me that long to learn that we parents should find, enjoy, and take advantage of them as much as humanly possible.

We might not get to go to a bar or to see a movie that isn't animated more than once every few years (Thomas and I went out just *two* times in five years), but finding fun in parenthood becomes easier as time passes and you gain a little something called perspective. Yes, even on the worst, most obnoxious days where that bright spot is no larger than a pin prick and you've got baby shit under your fingernails. (Don't pretend like it's never happened to you!)

Since the birth of my oldest, when I truly felt that I was at the end of my rope and simply couldn't handle any more asshattery, I began compiling folders comprised of carefully selected photos of naked bath times, dimply butt cheeks, bodies covered in stickers, and underwear on heads, to pull out at just the right moment when the boys get older. Like, oh, you know, their first dates, prom . . . maybe even engagement parties—but what about *now*? All of the above are still (hopefully) *many* years away, and karma is a slow ass bitch when it comes to payback for the evil shit the kids have done up until this point, but my arsenal is becoming stocked and these kids aren't even in double-digit ages yet. I was and am *always* in need of some instant gratification, and that is right at the tip of your fingers. I have a list of many of these insta-happy little things that I keep in the dark corners of my mind for tantrum-y butthole kid moments. I keep them there so I can think about them during these harrowing times and not go all Mommy Dearest up in this bitch.

Yes, my child, continue to freak out, because I know eventually the time will come where I will make a dessert your picky ass doesn't like, and you will refuse to eat it. Since I have already prepared it for consumption, it shall be mine. *All* mine! Sure, my tiny-terror, run around the yard screaming like you just escaped from prison while I cringe, waiting for you to inevitably bust your ass, which will create a booboo that I will be the one to have to deal with as you scream directly into my face, for I know this will only make it so that you sleep better and earlier tonight.

It's all about turning the negatives into positives! Not the easiest reality to accept, but while it sounds like super obnoxious Suzy Sunshine–type bullshit, it really does work on those days where you'd love nothing more than to be kidnapped by some old weird-beard and stashed in an underground tunnel for a couple of years, just so the only person around to annoy you is yourself.

While I'll admit there's nothing quite like the sound of a child belly-laughing, there are many other things that come pretty close. They may not make your teeth rot out of your head from absolute sweetness, but Mommy always said too much sugar is bad for you anyway. My personal favorite? Screams. That's right, I said screams! Not the hurt, hungry, tired, annoying, or—for no reason at all, just to be obnoxious screams—definitely not. I'm nutty, not completely off my rocker! Give me a little credit here. This road to parental acceptance is not always pretty.

Screams are my absolute, hands down, favorite of all the little things to enjoy, revel, and partake in. They should not be looked down at through the nostrils—for causing them is not mean, harsh, or cruel—it is life. In my opinion, it is best we teach our kids the fun you can have while your heart is pounding by scaring the balls off them. Not literally or anything, 'cause then I couldn't have grandbabies, but figuratively, absolutely *yes*.

I'm not suggesting forcing the poor things into a haunted house meant for grown adults and scarring them for life as a bloody clown chases them with a machete down dark corridors, or doing what *my* mom did and locking me upstairs in our house alone while slamming doors and flicking lights on and off telling little six-year-old me that if I went to the bathroom alone, Candyman would get me. This caused the "you're *ruining* my life, Mom!" conspiracy to start early and go much deeper than simple public embarrassment via white tube socks during my formative years and forcing me to eat beef flavored sawdust meatloaf. I can laugh about it *now*, but I know all my aversions started with Candyman. I don't want to scar my children for life . . . I just want to make them tinkle a little.

To this day, I *still* feel bad about taking the kids into the Halloween store one year and watching the pure unbridled terror spread across Parker's face within the first twenty seconds. The poor kid felt a fear so intense that his entire body froze, and he couldn't even make a sound as a giant fake spider lunged at him as he walked by. Really, that was all Thomas's fault, and I have the sneaking suspicion he did that shit on purpose.

The type of scaring I'm talking about is the good ol' "hide behind the door, jump out, and yell boo!" kind. I'm trying to make them shriek and then maybe giggle, not need years of intensive therapy. Oh, to watch them jump and flail their arms like wacky waving arm flailing inflatable tube men because I got them *so* good, and then break into a fit of laughter once they realize it was me and no one is going to devour them—there's not much better than that. I don't know what in the world makes it so damn funny to scare the crap out of a kid—it just *is*. Just like peanut butter and chocolate go together perfectly—these unions of awesome simply cannot be explained with mere words. You just have to get your ass behind a door, wait for your sweet, innocent, unsuspecting child to walk by, and pounce.

As sad as it is to watch children grow so quickly, we have to accept that there is only so long we can prank the shit out of them before they get old enough to start swinging on us . . . or God forbid doing it back, and *worse*! Soooooo much worse. You've seen the shows; the super pranks that I am positive are the leading cause of worry lines in parents' faces. Most of them don't even give out prizes for making mommy's bladder leak after leaving gigantic plastic bugs in her bed, or falling flat on the floor after someone hiding behind shower curtains with a Michael Myers mask on jumped out with a frickin' chainsaw. Oh, it's gonna happen, like it or not. Since we know this fate is inevitable, we learn that we must take advantage of this short window. I'm smashing through that mofo like the Kool-Aid Man. Oh yeah!

Any time I get them so good they fall backward, I'm reminded of not only being tortured with Candyman, but the tube socks, and the giant hair, and how it seemed as though my mom went out of her way to embarrass the shit out of me with what she wore and the things she said and did. I get the distinct feeling that wasn't who she actually was, but that it was all an elaborate hoax; a way to have fun by horrifying me with fear, food, and fashion. It's ingenious! Well played, Mom. Very well played, indeed. Even though I *still*, to this day, refuse to walk into a bathroom if the light is off, I can *finally* laugh at all the ways my parents embarrassed and horrified me growing up because I realize just how much *fun* it is. Now *that* is fucking terrifying!

CHAPTER **29**

TGIM: THANK GOD IT'S FRICKIN' MONDAY!

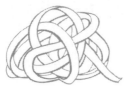

WHEN I WAS NINETEEN, I landed my first "real" job. I'd done a cornucopia of things already; customer service, pizza delivery, waiting tables—but finally, I was a working girl. No, not in the red light district on a corner. Geez! I had my own desk, set hours, and paid vacation; awesome, right? I hated every single solitary minute of it. The *only* upside, other than sick days I could use when I wasn't sick, was weekends off. Two whole days of not waking up early or dealing with menopausal bosses who insisted on keeping the entire office five degrees below freezing because they were having monstrous hot flashes. No more working on Saturday nights while my friends went out and partied. Yay!

Every Sunday I could already feel Monday digging her claws into me for another five days of hell; and every week I would look forward to Fridays and scream TGIF at the top of my lungs when it finally arrived. It was my shiny beacon of hope that this desk job wasn't going to drain all the life out of me. Friday! My savior!

The death of Friday was a bitter pill to swallow once I had kids to take care of. I'd still get all worked up because it was finally the weekend, which traditionally, in my mind, was a relaxing thought. Automatically my brain went to my happy place: Relief! Relax! Rejoice! Only to be awoken early on a Saturday morning to do the exact same things as the previous five days . . . only now I had a third whiny human to deal with: the husband.

My already worn out and confused Mommy Brain didn't know how to process this. For twenty-three years, the weekend was my break, and now, suddenly, it was even *more* exhausting than Monday through Friday? When do I get a break then? Do I even *get* one? I was less than pleased to learn that the answer to this question was a technical and resounding no. To this day, I have not fully accepted that, but the text messages I frequently get on the rare occasion that I am out of the house without kids—usually getting the grays *they* gave me covered up—from my husband asking repeatedly when I'll be back suggest that I should.

It seemed that all hope was lost. I had finally accepted the physical *and* mental changes that parenthood had on my life; things that are considered "sacrifices" by others didn't even get a second thought. I *chose* this "job" and everything that came along with it, but let's be real here—even if it's your dream job, you need time away. Time to recoup, recharge, and restock on a thing we like to call patience (a rare commodity in the parenting world).

You need time to just be *you*; without deadlines, assignments, or your obnoxious children screeching at you through the gap under the bathroom door. It's truly amazing what one trip alone to the bathroom can do for a parent's grip on sanity. When? How? This simply did not seem like a possibility, what with Parker, who made it nearly impossible for even me—his beloved mother only trying to do the best for him (to get him to eat)—mommy paranoia set in strong. Combine the fear of my child starving to death in the span of a few hours (yes, I know how ridiculous that sounds in retrospect), no one willing to watch the terrible twosome other than my incessantly texting husband, and a lack of funds or desire to go somewhere and sit in silence where I would only think about all of the above until I drove myself crazy enough to give up and go home, and my fate had been sealed *for* me. My breaks would only come in the form of the hours in which the boys actually slept.

In some ways, the isolation wasn't so bad. Far less drama occurred when the only people I interacted with on a daily basis couldn't even wipe their own asses. I far prefer the freak out over a missing stuffed animal than who is sleeping with who, so and so said this or that, or did you hear?! No. I didn't. Just assume I didn't from here on out. In a way, though, I missed it. Not being a part of the drama—oh, *hell* no—but just being a part of life outside my own house. I had actually started looking forward to trips to the library on Saturdays simply because it got me out in the "real" world. Would it *ever* change?

Yes. The answer is yes. The answer is a magical word consisting of six wonderful letters. One I used to dread, but now holds a completely different meaning to me: school!

I won't lie, overprotective mommy-me was sad about carting the OG of my uterus off to school for the first week. I missed him so much that the hours he was gone were miserable . . . and then I snapped the fuck out of it. What the hell was I thinking? Not only did someone else other than yours truly have to put up with his bullshit all day, but it's actually *quiet* in here! It had been so long since I'd only had one kid in this house that I'd forgotten just how peaceful it was. Actually, I don't think I ever really realized it in the first place. It was like going from an Ozzy concert to the Lilith Fair. I didn't know what the hell I'd do with myself. Sleep? Cry tears of joy?

The tables had turned from the life I once knew. While I love spending time with my family, and the weekend is the only real chance we get to do that for more than an hour (due to Thomas's work schedule during the week), come Sunday morning I find myself anxious for Monday to hurry the hell up, just like I once felt anxious for Friday to end. I'm still having trouble believing it myself, but I actually look *forward* to the dreaded Monday. That poor day really does get a bad rap.

Realizing Monday was my new Friday made for an extremely strange moment in my life.

Now I understand why my parents were always so excited for the first day of school. It's like an early Christmas gift! I always assumed it was just because they liked to see me suffer. Unlike my other realizations about my parental units, this time I learned that I was *totally right*! Hell yes, my parents enjoyed sending me away! Can you blame them? Kids, as much as we love them, are frickin' psycho! If the only break we can get is school? We embrace it with wide open arms! I also understand that things like Spring Break, Winter Break, and, of course, the big mamma-jamma Summer Break are nothing more than cruel play-on-words.

Oh, they're a break alright; break a plate, or a glass, or an obnoxious toy, or my damn sanity!

I'm thinking instead of getting Holden's present and future teachers some smelly-good lotion or some kind of hideous ceramic piece of junk that he would want to pick out for their end-of-the-year gifts, I'm going to get them a gift card to the liquor store.

They deserve it.

CHAPTER 30

No, but seriously. go the fuck to sleep!

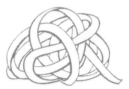

My parents loved mornings. After all I've learned about them through my own experiences, I am unsure if that was to further torture me or because I forced them to change. Adapting is a trait all humans should develop, but some things should just be considered cruel. Like the hours between sleep and 5 a.m.

In no shape, form, or creative stretch of the imagination could I *ever* be considered a morning person. This is another one of those things that I don't think can be learned or picked up over time; either you are born liking mornings or hating them. I am only a few steps under pure unbridled hatred. We have bad blood between us, me and the a.m. hours.

I can't completely blame my mom's affinity for early Saturday morning wake-ups to clean my room, or even how much I detested her barging into my room and rudely awakening me with song for just how much I loathe the wee hours of the morning. Did I mention my Mom was absolutely tone deaf? Or perhaps that was on purpose. . . . Anyway, not even thirteen years of school wake-ups before any human should rise, or months of choosing to get up at four in the morning to work an hour of overtime, could change my mind.

Also, if we're being brutally honest here, mornings make me downright nauseous. No, I'm not baking a baby, unless you consider "new life" to be what my ass angrily gives birth to if I have to rise before even the sun has bothered to. I am *allergic* to mornings; I'm convinced of it. Don't argue with me in your head. Logic has no place here!

When I learned I was going to be a parent, I'd heard all about how I'd never get any restful sleep ever again (or for eighteen years, at least) and I laughed. I hated mornings so much, it simply *had* to be passed down to anything that spent nine months occupying my insides. It's science! And I thought to myself, if this thing isn't *born* hating mornings, it will *learn*! It's not that I want to sleep the entire day away, but if you ask me, if it's still dark outside, it's just unnatural to get out of bed and start the "day." That is nothing more than a sick joke.

I have found over time, while pretending to be a productive and responsible adult, that there are simply not enough hours in the day to get done everything that needs to be done, so going to bed early to be able to wake up less stabby with more time to get ready is not an option. Throw kids into the mix and there are only three words that I can find to describe the feeling accurately: we are tired!

I miss sleep, plain and simple. I miss it a lot. If I could just get back all the naps I refused as a child, that would be fan-fucking-tastic! As the years passed and the kids *still* insisted on annoying me out of sleep before Thomas's alarm for work pierced through the morning silence, I had sourly resolved that a fulfilling, refreshing slumber simply wasn't in the cards for me. Kids have no damn idea what they're missing! Nor do they care. Sigh.

Children are ambivalent to our suffering. It takes time to accept that, but it's true. No matter how much I moaned and groaned, tried to put them back to bed, threatened, maybe even cried, the kids would be up before seven o'clock every single morning without fail. With Holden, I thought I could outsmart him. I sacrificed my night "thank you cheezus the kid is *finally* asleep and I can relax" time to keep that sucker up late in hopes that I would wear his crazy ass out and maybe, possibly, *please for the love of all that is holy*, he would sleep in. Even if just for an hour! At that point, I was even willing to accept ten measly minutes.

I learned an important lesson that month: do not negotiate with those tiny terrorists. He not only did *not* sleep in, but the later I kept him up, the earlier he would rise the next morning. I was incensed! He was amused. And chipper. It was fucking irritating.

Once I finally got the kid to the age where it was possible to doze a little in the a.m. after he insisted on getting out of bed—*without* him dumping a bag of chips onto the living room floor and then doing an Irish clog dance on top of them (which actually made a very soothing crackling sound, believe it or not)—along came Parker. One kid might be relatively simple to ignore while you try to catch just a few extra minutes of sleep in hopes of becoming a slightly operational human being (or something that resembles one), but two was like a tag-team from hell. I now understood why some people described parenthood as being pecked to death by chickens.

I'd get one of them back to bed after he woke up tripping over and smashing absolutely everything in sight while stomping the floor like the fucking Hulk, and then the other would wake up. How could anyone sleep through what sounded like the apocalypse? Once I got *that* one back to bed, his crying from being woken up by the first had somehow convinced numero uno that we were all getting up, and he'd get back out of his bed. By the third round of this bullshit—if I actually managed to crawl my own ass into my own warm and comfortable bed and close my eyes—they'd pop right back open. Awake. *Wide* awake.

It was time to accept my fate: sleeping was not going to happen. And it wasn't even seven yet.

The day I realized there would be no more real sleeping in, that I could not train these buttholes to understand early morning hours are like the seventh circle of hell, was a very sad day in my history.

It had been a long time since I had come to terms with my new way of life as an unwilling morning person when it happened. I opened my eyes, which had not been forced or pried open once, and looked around. At first, I was in a complete panic. Why am I awake? Why isn't there any noise? Am I dreaming? Am I *dead*? I did not hear the familiar sounds of shrieking or smashing or whining, and *holy shit*—it was light outside! For the first time in years, I felt completely refreshed, well-rested, alert, even. So alert that upon realizing that this *never* happens, I shot out of bed, thinking I'd been abandoned by my family or that they'd been abducted by aliens.

No. . . . Thomas was right next to me, still asleep. I checked the kids' rooms, and they were still sleeping, too. Then I looked at the clock. It MUST be four in the frickin' a.m., and I am completely delusional right now, thinking it's light outside when really it's the middle of the stupid ass night. The clock blinked in giant red numbers: 8:00 a.m. I silently happy-danced my ass back into my bedroom; we'd done it! We had all *actually* slept until the sun came up! Eight a.m. meant I actually slept in! Wait, what? Never in a million years did I think I would consider eight o'clock to be "sleeping in," but parenthood does weird things to a person.

What did I do next? This isn't the Super bowl; I didn't yell "I'm going to Disney World!" That would be totally awesome, but no. I woke everyone else up to tell them. Fuck if they're gonna sleep later than me! Payback's a bitch!

CHAPTER 31

I'M A LYING LIAR WHO LIES OUT OF MY LYING LIAR HOLE

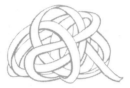

SOME PEOPLE MIGHT SAY I'M weird or loud, perhaps slightly paranoid or a little whiny. And by some people, I mean my family. I'm not able to truthfully deny any of the above, but if there is one thing I am *not*, it's a liar. I am brutally honest, even to a fault. Don't ask me if your ass looks fat in those pants if you don't want me to tell you that your crack resembles a black hole for denim. Alright, maybe I'm not *that* mean, but you will know not to wear those cracktacular pants in public ever again, that's for damn sure. My "beluga whale" mom would have been able to confirm this.

More times than I can count, I have had friends get mad at me when they come to me for advice and I tell them the truth. I blame the fact that I had kids before everyone else and thereby became the (cringe) Mom of the group, but I was still young enough to be asked about disgustingly embarrassing things without getting a lecture like they would from their *actual* giver of life. If all you want me to tell you is what you *want* to hear instead of my honest thoughts and feelings, I am not the one to come to. Stay far, far away from me. Or bribe me with brownies. I might be willing to glaze over the truth with lies as thick as delicious Krispy Kreme doughnut goop for brownies.

It's funny to think back on how totally clueless and wrong I was about all things parent-related. I joked when I saw kids on leashes and just thought it was the most awful and disrespectful thing you could ever do to your children. And *lazy*! Don't forget lazy! Come to find out (the hard way, of course) that some little shits just run. They run away and play hide-and-seek in clothing racks (but don't inform anyone that they're playing) or bolt at the first chance they get for no fucking reason at all, effectively shaving years off their poor parents' lives. It is just wiser and safer to bungee their asses to you than take the chance of allowing them to roam free. Take palm, smack against forehead repeatedly for not understanding it sooner. Some people hate when kids are referred to as experiments, but we have no damn idea what the hell we're doing! It's trial-and-error! It only takes one failed experiment of letting go of that clammy little hand and having their ass disa-fucking-ppear to say "Kid leashes? Hell *yes*, I get why!"

Parental laziness, it is not. What it *is*, is assholey childhood independence, and it is terrifying. I've yet to use a leash on either of my two, but I can't say it isn't tempting . . . like those brownies covered in glaze that you should bribe me with when you ask about those pants you're wearing that are two sizes too small.

When it came to Christmas, I wasn't sure what I was going to do, with me being all Honest Abe-ish. (Without the beard. I Nair that shit. Duh!) I didn't see the point in lying to my bratty kids by telling them that some creepy stranger was going to squeeze his enormous ass down our chimney and leave them presents that they earned because he'd been watching them day and night to monitor their behavior. Even worse would be telling them that the only way to appease the one called Santa Claus was to be good and to feed him milk and cookies. Why are we feeding this weirdo and not reporting him to the police?

To me, that sounded more like the plot to a B-rated horror film. Plus, this stalkery freak got credit for the shit *I* spent *my* money on? What the?? Shenanigans!

It really is true that there are some things in life you really can't even *begin* to understand until you have incubated a baby. You have to learn through experience and those pesky failed experiments (read: jacking up the first kid) that childhood is a very short period in life; one in which magic is *real*. Once you see that magic in your child's eyes, you think, "Eh, one little white lie won't hurt them!"

There's only so long that kids are gullible enough to believe in a magic elf who delivers gifts via sled pulled by flying reindeer or a bunny that shits delicious jellybeans. I couldn't *not* let them experience that! Even if I hate lying, this is a special exception to my strict rule.

That one allowance was at the very top of a slippery slope, my friends; a very slippery slope indeed!

It didn't take long after opening that door that I realized glossing over the truth made life a hell of a lot easier with whiny little humans running around. I still don't condone being blatantly dishonest, but when it comes to little kids, sometimes the truth just ain't gonna cut it. They won't understand, or it's too complicated, or it would start an infuriating marathon of "Why?"s when you just don't have the mental energy to answer them all. A few teensy tiny white lies aren't so bad!

While potty training Holden, once he realized there were bathrooms in places other than home, he *insisted* on using all of them—every single one. If he even *saw* a bathroom sign, I'd hear "I have to pee!" come out of his mouth faster than a baby can shit in a brand new diaper. There's not much more frustrating than taking a child to a public bathroom and getting nothing more than a little drip drip. Of course, this is *after* getting them undressed from the waist down, plopping them on the seat—trying to make sure they don't touch the wretched thing with their hands because of the disgusting amount of butt-germs that could be living there—all while squatting into a horribly uncomfortable position to keep them steady. All done! Are you kidding me?! I mean, thank you for informing me you needed to go, good job for not pissing yourself out in the open, but are you fucking *kidding* me with this shit? That's *it*?! After the sixth time this nonsense happened, I had had about enough.

The next time those beady little toddler eyes caught sight of a bathroom? "Oh no, honey. It's broken!"

Sometimes I wouldn't even let it get that far. No, there is no bathroom here so don't even ask because you *just* went. You are not an animal and you do not need to mark your territory! Sure, it might sound selfish; maybe even lazy. I even had many sharp pangs of the dreaded mommy-guilt. You know what, though? It saved us a buttload of time while out. We don't have much of that as it stands without someone melting down and having to retreat back to home base. Like I said, it's a slippery slope. White lies are nothing but a gateway drug to lies of total convenience.

Pangs of mommy-guilt soon gave way to relaxation and the stalling of the tinsel-colored hair sprouting from my head. I'm not embarrassed, and I don't even regret any of it. I'll admit it right here and right now. Fast food joint play-places may be what children's dreams are made of, but I don't care. Call me a dream crusher if you must. My bad, I just have an aversion to OPPG: Other People's Poo Germs. My kids are not getting smeared in them. Fun? No. A closed plastic tube full of boogery, pants-crapping, inefficient butt-wiping, tiny humanoid heathens who crawl on their hands and knees and then proceed to pop those hands into their crusty mouths without washing them, writhing around together and spreading that (literal) shit around like warm butter?

"I'm so sorry, honey! You're just not tall enough yet!"
One year later?

"Sorry honey! Your brother just isn't tall enough and he will scream if you get to play and he doesn't! It just wouldn't be fair! Maybe next time!"

They may never grasp it (oh *please* don't let them catch on), but there won't ever be a next time. "Next time" really just means "Never! I just want you to leave me alone so I shall subdue you with this miniscule lie!" "Next time," Parker will miraculously have *just* gone through a five-inch growth spurt. Hopefully, Holden won't know how to accurately measure height by then.

I don't see it as being mean, or ridiculous, or just plain frigid and un-fun. I do an enormous amount of miserable crap for my kids that they think is awesome. OPPG is not one of them, and it never will be! If you didn't come out of my baby-maker, I don't want your poo on, near, or microscopically spread all over me or my kids. What's wrong with that? I ask you. If your answer isn't "Nothing!" you're wrong!

I say things taste good even if I find them gross to get my kids to eat them because nutrition is important. I didn't tell them what a vagina is yet because I know they'd shout it in public, even if that means they occasionally comment that I have a "weird pecker." Ixnay on the eriod-pay! We don't discuss Aunt Flo or the menstrual cycle yet; that is on a need-to-know basis. Plus, they're never even going to be cursed with it! One time of my tampon loudly being referred to as a "rabbit tail" was more than enough to convince me to keep the truth to myself for a while longer. If I just don't feel like sharing a beverage or hiding in the bathroom and drinking it on the toilet, I tell them it has alcohol in it. Instant win!

We parents all have our own strange methods, rules, admissions, and retractions, and we all have our legitimate (to us) reasons for them. Some might even make sense to *other* people! It's called adapting, and it's pretty frickin' amazing once you figure out that it might add the years back to your life that your kids chipped off.

Telling them a restaurant they love is closed to avoid eating there when I've asked for suggestions, however, I don't have a good excuse for. They just have disgusting taste, and even if I have no idea where I personally want to dine, I will still shoot down their ideas. I will also ninja roll into their rooms to replace their nasty little baby teeth with change and tell them that the creeptacular human body part trafficker Tooth Fairy did it. No shame whatsoever!

There was even a time I took their obnoxious talking Elmo, and with my best voice impression, made it say terrifying things to the kids in hopes they would be too scared to ever play with it again. It worked. I nearly shat myself, I was so overjoyed! I fucking *hate* that furry freak. I know he's educational, and I guess if I narrow my eyes he's kind of cute . . . but how can you like someone who talks about themselves in the third person?

I'd become a habitual liar. Maybe I should have felt guilty; I was lying through my teeth to sweet, innocent little *children*, the horror! But I wasn't feeling guilty. Not even a little bit! How's that for accepting my inner-mom? just good that liars' pants don't really catch on fire or I'd have third-degree burns on my ass so painful I may never poop again. I guess then I'd finally have a real excuse to avoid visiting every public restroom known to man.

CHAPTER 32

WHEN IN DOUBT, BLAME THE SPROUT

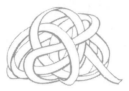

ALL OF THE BITCHING, MOANING, and complaining about needing sleep, a break, five quiet seconds, never getting to go anywhere, or being so stir crazy that my skull is going to explode if I don't get the hell out of the house doesn't change the fact that sometimes, I just don't *really* want to go anywhere. Remember when we used to stay up all night and called it "fun"? That shit's hilarious to me now . . . in a not-so hilarious way.

I have always been a woman of my word. If I say I'm going to be somewhere or do something—I'm there, and I do it; and I loathe excuses. When you toss a whining, obnoxious, possibly sick-ish, bratty little kid or two into the mix—plus a severe lack of sleep—it makes it difficult to be that word-keeping woman *all* the time. You hope and pray and cross your fingers, toes, testicles, and nipples (if they hang that low) for the skies to open up and rain out these plans you made so that you don't have to be the asshole who cancels at the last second.

A freak blizzard! A plague of locusts! A truck full of bowling balls overturning and shutting down the only way to get to the place you are supposed to be! Of course, *none* of that ever happens. So what to do you do? Do you just suck it up and go? Maybe . . . but there comes a time in every parent's life where they use their sweet, innocent, little child to get out of a commitment.

This admission may not make me popular with my friends, but I know you're over there silently nodding in agreement. I know, it's hard to come clean about what your kid has morphed you into, but it's better late than never! Friends: if you feel the butthurt taking hold—don't even play—I *know* you've done it to me, too! Yes, I'm *so* sure little precious suddenly has the sniffles for the past *two* things I've invited you to. Don't even try that shit. We all know what's really going on here.

If our kid has a little random sniffle or is in a rotten ass mood, we could *absolutely* still take them out. The fact is that we simply don't *want* to. Who wants to deal with that hot ass mess in public where everyone is glaring at you for interrupting their good time with your loudmouth spawn that won't stop whining? Sorry, friends! We'd love to come, but the poor kid isn't feeling so well. Sure would hate to ruin your plans with my wailing product of procreation! It's for the best, honestly. You should be thanking me!

Kids are the best excuses ever invented, er, created. And to think they came from something as dumb as genitalia!

We love the shit out of them, but we blame them for everything from weight gain to wrinkles, gray hairs, floppy no-no bits, and getting out of our second cousin's third wedding to the dude she met in the Craigslist "Missed Connections" section. It might not be anything to brag about, but after the floppy no-no's and constant dangling over the brink of sanity, don't we deserve a perk? Yeah, yeah—love, affection, and the unbreakable and unmatched bond between parent and child. I'm not talking about that junk. You should know me better by now!

Sometimes we parents are greedy and we want more than that love and emotion stuff. Don't sit over there shaking your head. The day will come when your child has a slight case of mud-butt and you really didn't want to go somewhere anyway, nor do you want to have to go through the horror of changing their ass repeatedly outside the comfort of your own home. Even though you could totally do it with very little effort, you will use that poor poopy child as an excuse not to go. Shame on you!! I'm kidding! I'm on your side! Some days I wonder how I even manage to get myself dressed, let alone two crapping kids. Getting out of the house? I try to avoid that if at all possible. Yes, that means taking advantage of my own unsuspecting children. This even means faking a case of mud-butt from time to time. I can feel it coming! I swear! Lil' dude had a wet fart that just couldn't be trusted and now we're stuck in the house. Oh, darn!

Yes, I know I'm a terrible person. I can live with that.

You know, one of these days, the kids are going to wise up and ask why I get so excited when they tell me they don't feel well.

"But Mommy, don't you hate it when I'm sick? Don't you love me?" they'd say.

"Of course I love you, sweetie, but today I love being able to lounge on this couch just a *little* bit more!"

CHAPTER 33

THE POO WHISPERER

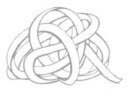

EVEN THOUGH I'D BEEN A parent for years, there was one question I could never seem to find the answer to: Who is "they"? You know, the "they" who say this and that; the "they" who try to teach you important lessons. How can you trust someone as vague as a "they"? To this day, I don't exactly know who "they" are, but sometimes these ominous know-all beings really hit the nail on the head. *They* say "what doesn't kill you makes you stronger," and you think, well, *duh*. I don't really know if by saving a penny I've earned it, or if two in the hand is worth one in the bush (mostly because I have no earthly idea what that even means) but sometimes, the age-old sayings really do ring true for your life.

Numerous times in my late teens, I was warned by those older and seemingly wiser (Ahem, parents!) that you "never *really* know someone until you live with them." Apparently dear old Mom and Dad subscribed to the same newsletter as the mysterious "they," because none of them ever specified just how intimately that would be, or that it would multiply times a thousand when your roommates were created with your very own private parts. I probably wouldn't have listened if "they" or my folks *had* told me, but that's beside the point!

From the time I moved out on my own until the day I moved in with the man who would become my husband, I spent a lot of time dealing with a wide array—some might even call it a buttload—of disgusting ass roommates from all walks of life. Each with all different levels of hygiene. I can *still* smell some of them. There was the forty-something drunken stoner "golf pro" who would shock me out of a restful slumber by blasting psychedelic shit music from the seventies at two in the morning—one time, so loud that I thought he was having a massive party, only to storm out of my room in my fugly ass pajamas to find him sitting in the middle of the den by himself, swaying back and forth and reeking of beer. Yeah, I didn't stay in that house for very long. Oh, and then there was the twenty-year-old mama's boy and his anti-deodorant best friend from high school who never showered. Those two butt-buddies spent every night all night together with their online role-playing games. That ended because mama didn't like me, and apparently I was corrupting poor lil' precious by bringing alcohol into the house. Alcohol that was his. I also had female roommates. Once. They were *that* bad.

Although I got to know many (what should have been) confidential details I never had *any* desire to discover, and after prolonged co-habitations, learned to expect weird shit like late-night bed smoking, sitting on top of fridges, and what someone smells like after not having bathed for . . . possibly ever, I only took away one important lesson from it all. That whole "older and wiser" thing "they" say? It is remarkably accurate, even though I didn't want it to be. I'm stubborn like that. I might be willing to admit that to "they," them, any of the people I had the unfortunate experience to live with, or my parents, if they'd all promise not to de-age by about ten years and do the "Told ya so!" dance, but I know how hard that is to resist. Instead, I just accepted that the "best friend" I was living with was best taken in small doses (or not at all), moved out, and swore never to have roommates again.

Finding another human who you can *actually* tolerate being in a confined space with for a prolonged period of time only occurs once in a blue moon. When it does, it's so exciting that occasionally what happens is you take on a third tenant. Poof! It's like magic! They won't run up your electric bill or sit in your living room blasting shit music at ungodly hours of the night, but they *do* have the tendency to overstay their welcome and never fucking pay a single dime of rent.

If you haven't figured it out, I'm talking about a uterine subletter. A baby. My husband is the only one I could actually stand living with for longer than a year. I don't think I need to elaborate on how babies are made.

I can't be sure if it's some kind of strange, undiscovered scientific or psychic link, or maybe just the shared chromosomes and genetics, but once I got used to the intermittent "Holy fuck, what am I doing? Why are you crying? What do you want? *What's wrong?* I'm going crazy! I don't understand!" emotional breakdowns that parenthood is kind enough to supply, something in my sleep-deprived brain clicked. I just *got it*.

Although I'm positive it didn't happen easily, it felt like, out of nowhere, I knew what sounds and which cries required attention and which ones only necessitated a call from my comfortable position on the couch (which is about as rare and elusive as Big Foot). There is an obviously glazed-over look in a child's eyes when they are tired but insisting they aren't that, somehow, I'd never been able to pick up on before. But now I was aware of it. Things just seemed to be falling into place; things that confused the shit out of me before became second nature.

Life is pretty good when you don't spend over half of it not having a single solitary clue what the crap is going on around you.

This new power of mine (which I like to think is the third eye other moms are constantly referring to when threatening their young) came in handy for a lot more than just practical uses around the house. I am still undecided on whether the strength of this power is a blessing or a curse. It gets put to use when dealing with my two long-term roommates (a.k.a. children). They don't really get along all that well, probably because they didn't know each other prior to moving in, but they are so much alike. You would swear they are related! This extreme compatibility can also lead to a constant butting of heads only worsened when trapped within the confines of one home. I guess they *could* leave, but the freeloaders don't have licenses so I have to chauffer them everywhere. The nerve!

Even as much as they claim not to like one another, they are *always* together. I dare even call their relationship "inseparable," but don't tell them I said so. They'd deny it. The best toys (judging by their attachments to them) can be found hidden away upstairs in their bedrooms, which means more often than not, they are up there playing. I regularly welcome this reprieve from the assault on my ears that a level of plywood and plaster muffles on the rare afternoon they leave me downstairs by my lonesome.

Sadly, it is short-lived, because they *always* end up fighting over something ridiculously stupid. Who has the blue car that the other got for their birthday? It's the end of the frickin' world, y'all! Even though they both got the Same. Exact. One. This renders their reasoning for devolving into a slap-fight moot, but that doesn't matter to them one bit. These fights usually end in one of them stomping down the stairs so that they can tattle on the other. Lucky me.

It was during one of these obnoxiously pointless fights when the one who had decided to be the tattler for the day got halfway down the stairs, and without him even saying a word, I yelled "Holden, do *not* tattle! I don't want to hear any tattling!" There was a short pause, and then the footsteps retreated back up the stairs. I had known who was coming to tattle by the sound of their footsteps alone!

Usually the kid would argue with me until he was blue in the face: "But . . . but *he* . . . But . . ." *But* . . . I think he was so shocked the first time this happened that, for once in his life, he was totally speechless.

"Oh my God! Mommy really *can* see everything!"

Cue evil laugh. Thank you, third eye.

We all know I can't, but if the kids think I can? That's a *major* blessing. I can even tell by the way they're standing if they need to restock the lake with brown trout. It has saved me from having to spray poo out of what would have been destroyed pairs of underwear *many* times. *Major* blessing! The same goes for my husband; after so many years of marriage, there's not much left that Thomas and I keep from each other. The man has watched me shoot two children out of my vagina while speaking in tongues like Linda Blair in *The Exorcist* and still apparently finds me attractive. What is there left to be shy about after that?

For me, it's farting. I can't stand it, yet somehow I ended up with the gassiest man on the planet who, in turn, impregnated me with the two gassiest children on the planet. My house is constantly filled with the noxious ass-fumes of my long-term roommates. He knows I hate it, and I've asked him repeatedly to go at *least* out of ear and nose range before he blows, but instead of listening, he bombs the room and blames it on the kids. This rubbed off on the wee ones, and now no one is safe from having the stench permeating the room pinned on them. Not even me, the non-farter. That all ended after lunch one weekend.

We make it a point when everyone is home to eat meals together as one big, dysfunctional family unit. Conversation ranges from talking about the day, school, work, to whatever the hell else comes to mind (and anything is possible with children). Even with the choice in topics we have, even on a busy day where there's not enough time to talk about everything, even on the days where we're running so far behind schedule that we don't talk at all and all we have time for is to cram food into our faces, one thing *always* happens.

Someone farts.

At the table!

While we're eating!

Are you nasty asses *kidding* me? You can't hold it? Squeak it out so I don't hear it so once the stench assaults my nose, I wonder if perhaps it's my own funk? Leave the room so that my meal isn't ruined by the smell of rotten food coming out of your rear end? Sensing my building level of rage, they panic. Fingers started flying, pointing at the nearest person while yelling "he did it!" in order to avoid my wrath. Yes, this includes my husband.

Farting ruined every single meal in my house for the better part of a decade, until the day I'd had enough of the fart-blame game. I don't know what came over me; I cannot tell you what the hell I was thinking, or even if I was thinking at all, but while the fingers were pointing and the blame was flying, I took a big ol' whiff of the flatulence-filled air. I then looked right at my family and pointed my finger at the guilty party.

"Don't lie, Thomas. *You* did it!"

As capable as the man is, one thing he cannot do is lie. He hung his head and accepted ownership of the putrid kitchen atmosphere. Kid crap smells like crap; husband crap smells like he's rotting from the inside. Sorry, Thomas; there's just no fooling me anymore.

That's right. I'm admitting the unthinkable: I know my family so well that I can identify them by the smells of their farts. Even in my wildest dreams (or nightmares), I never imagined that something like this would not only be true, but that it would come in handy as a mom. It wasn't that far in the past that I would have been positively mortified about what I'd done, and for good reason! My cheerleadery Supermom power was fart-sniffing? *Seriously*? But . . . other moms got the quiet-yet-terrifying voice, craftiness, morning perkiness, and being able to tell when household items are being dumped in the toilet without ever hearing a sound, and I got *fart-sniffing*? I'd say it's not fair, but since I became well-versed in the art of being wrong, I knew it was best just to relax and accept the crazy. I was a Mom Scout and this was my brand new shiny merit badge! Like a deck of cards, parenthood will often deal us hands full of jokers and expect us to make good use of them.

You're over there cringing, aren't you? Being able to know who farted by simply sniffing the air isn't so repulsively revolting once you realize that no one in your household can ever successfully blame their fart on anyone else *ever* again! It's about time the dogs stopped taking so much of the heat for the humans here. More importantly, no one would ever be able to blame *me* for their farts in public again. Try playing off a loud wet fart when all the fingers are pointing at you. Kids are assholes. And they use their assholes against us. Well, not anymore!

I should update my resume with the title The Poo Whisperer; I'm also fluent in toddler-ese. I am positive that these *must* be marketable skills in the workforce today.

CHAPTER 34

HOW TO WEAR A BOOGER LIKE A BADGE OF HONOR

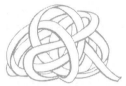

ONE THING I NEVER WANTED to be was the parent with what I called "the grubby kid."

You know the kind I'm talking about. Your eyes are happily scanning through a public place when suddenly they freeze on the face of a child and it shocks you two steps backwards. They have some kind of food remnants crusted around their mouths, or maybe it's dirt. Or shit. It could be shit for all you know! They just look to be a hot ass mess and you have to wonder how they ever got out of the house looking that nasty. Then I find that I kind of hate myself for being that judgy-mom who everyone loathes and who needs a swift chop to the baby-maker. At the same time, I swore I would be a crud-dictator so no one would ever wonder that about my kids or my parenting.

No crud would ever get out of this door! Leaving this house was like trying to board a plane, with multiple security checks to get through. One for clothes, one for corners of mouths, another for possible dangling nose-gremlins and, of course, the dreaded and cringe-worthy eye boogers. Yes, I am and always have been fully aware that boys are disgusting little creatures often defined by the expression "noise with dirt on it" but, damnit, they were going to look as clean and sparkly as humanly possible if I had anything to do with it! I wasn't going for *Twilight* levels of glittering beauty, here. I was anal, not unrealistic.

Keeping them clean was nearly a full-time job in and of itself, because damn if being lower to the ground didn't have some kind of magnetic pull on things like mud and grass and food I wasn't even aware they had been eating in the first place. I guess if we're being sincere, sometimes it wasn't even food they were eating. The whole eye in the back of the head/third eye threat needs to become legitimately real at this point. We parents have to defy science and nature to pop one of those bitches out of our skulls if we don't want a toddler who looks like they've channeled a Woodstock mud-person.

I don't mean to pat myself on the back or anything, but judging by all the compliments I've gotten on the boys' clothing over the years, I think I was doing an impeccable job of keeping them bright and shiny like a new car. The smell has never been something I could control, but at least they *appeared* to be clean, and that's what's important, right? I did such a good job at de-gunking the boys' clothes, in fact, that I *completely* forgot about my own. Who has time to think about that when there are mud puddles and ant hills to avoid. (Seriously. Ant hills. WTF?)

It's not like I spent time rolling around in dirt and needed to keep myself in check like an adolescent. I care about how I look, even after the night when someone who shall remain nameless (Parker) woke me up fourteen times. I bathe. I scrub. I use tissues and I've had more than twenty years' worth of experience wiping my own ass. I don't even like dirt. If you're not yet convinced, I wasn't wearing pajamas or yoga pants *and* I brushed my hair. I was golden!

Out the door I went with a little spring in my step. It wasn't until I was out in public, visiting the bathroom for the fifth time because *someone*—again not naming any names (Parker!!!)—had the bladder of a fucking mosquito, that I caught a glimpse of the back of my nice, clean (or so I thought) shirt, and something caught my eye. Something green-ish. What could that be? Wracking my brain, I knew that—with reasonable certainty—I hadn't eaten anything green that day. Shit, I'm not even flexible enough to reach all the way back there anymore, so I knew automatically it couldn't have been put there by me.

Closer and closer I crept to the smudged up bathroom mirror that teen girls seem so fond of photographing themselves in these days, and that is when the source of the mysterious green smudge dawned on me. There I was, so *touched* that my sweet little child asked me for a hug out of nowhere, and even let it linger longer than usual. At the time, I was so overwhelmed with parental love that I didn't care why, or if there even was a reason at all. I accepted that hug without a second thought—who wouldn't? There never needs to be a reason for a hug! Now I knew the horrible truth: it was just an excuse to wipe a giant honking snot-wad on my shirt.

I sighed deeply. This ain't my first rodeo. After a failed attempt to remove the wad of booger attached to the fabric, I shrugged my shoulders, said "Fuck it!" and continued on with my day. The looks? Who cares!

Early on, we birth-givers all learn the hard (read: wet) way that there is *no* point in changing unless you are so soaked in baby pee or chunky puke that it's dripping from your clothing. There were even days that, after the fourth outfit change for both me and the human upchuck-bucket, even a little poo could stay. It didn't even matter if it made zero sense that my kid looked spotless while I looked like a dumpster full of rotten vegetables had exploded on me.

After going through that times two, one booger was *nothing*! It sure as hell beat the alternatives. I am okay with being a human napkin if it means we avoid *ever* having one of them flicking that boog and hitting some stranger right in the face. Not that I'd know from personal experience or anything . . . but I'd imagine that would be pretty embarrassing. Should I be ashamed that one of my most uttered phrases these days is "just go ahead and wipe your hands on me"? Because I'm not. I wear their snot and mouth crusties like badges of honor. More mom merit badges! Woohoo! Sometimes they're even color-coordinated with my outfits. I'm so stylish!

CONCLUSION

Let's wrap it up! unless you're trying to get pregnant . . .

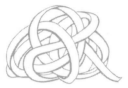

NOT LONG AGO, AS I was running up to the school for afternoon pick-up, I was referred to as Holden's Mom instead of my first or last name for the very first time. It was so strange; almost like an out-of-body experience. Even after six years, all the firsts, sicknesses, battles, tantrums, tears, and turds, being called Mom by strangers, and Mommy by two little boys is still surreal. I have *two* humans who I created and grew inside my guts living in my house, looking at me, and horror of all horrors, looking up *to* me. I'm not sure I'll ever get used to that.

Some days as I watch them chase each other around the yard screaming "Peanut butter sandwich!" for reasons I will probably never know or understand, I feel ten years older. Two kids; two *crazy,* possibly deranged kids. How the hell did that happen? I can't help but smile at those times, but even on the days that I could sell them on online for the best offer, I wouldn't. Not just because it's highly illegal and would get me thrown in jail, and if we're being honest, prison orange is not my color; it's more than that. It's also not *completely* because I know they'd be returned to me within the first hour and I'd have to refund the money I was planning on using to get Botox to rid my face of the worry lines they helped create on my forehead, but because *most* of the time they're pretty damn awesome. I'd miss the little shits if they were gone.

Who else would blame my farts on someone else when they knew it was me? Who else would announce that I was exorcising my anus to an entire public restroom full of people, or ask me why I have a "cotton tail like a bunny" when Aunt Flo is punching me in the uterus for a week? Who the hell else could I ever convince to use their adorable puppy eyes to beg their father for Taco Bell because I want it, but it's more likely to happen if they are the ones doing the asking because they are just so hard to say no to?

No one, that's who.

This whole book has been full of the ways that everything has changed since those two came crashing into my world and permanently affected me in ways that, no matter how unreal or weird it feels, or how hard I kicked and screamed, make my status as Mom undeniable. Sure, I may never be able to look at certain hunky actors the same way again because all I can hear when they open their mouths is the voice they lent to one of my kid's favorite animated films. I may never again actually get to see a movie those actors are in that doesn't have a G rating and makes me die a little inside, and I have accepted that to the point where I tell people to go ahead and spoil new releases for me.

Maybe I'll never pee alone again, know what sleeping past seven thirty in the morning feels like, or get an ice cream cone to myself. It might be true that I nearly had a coronary when I had to trade in my sedan for a larger vehicle and saw it listed on my registration as a "wagon," and the most exciting part of my days may be walking down the driveway to get the mail, but as much as I cringed at the thought of being called Mom . . . I don't *totally* hate it.

I know how many times I said, "I'll never be *that* kind of mom." I can't even count them all, but I'm pretty sure the number is up in the thousands by now. We all know the kind I mean without even having to say it because they always end up getting portrayed on TV as the frumpy, uptight, overbearing, crazy ladies who are always two seconds away from snapping and having CPS called on them. It's a stereotype, an ugly one at that, but it had to come from somewhere, didn't it? A tiny morsel of truth, perhaps? The kind I fought so hard against turning into. The kind I denied any resemblance to because all of that bologna was what really had me believing that *mom* was a bad word, and *no way* would that be me! *That* kind of mom? I'll never be that kind of mom! I'll be a way better parent than those crazies on TV! The words bounce around in my mostly vacant head now that my remaining brain cells have been melted away by years of Spongebob and Dora the stupid Explorer.

I'll never be the kind of mom who makes people annoyed or disgusted with my tales of diaper changes gone awry or leaky nipples. I'll never act like the world should revolve around my kid and everything else is insignificant in comparison. I'll never be the kind of mom who whines about the UPS driver ringing the doorbell during nap time as though they should *automatically* know a child inside is *trying* to sleep. I'll never be the kind of mom who carries around hand sanitizer and goes completely batshit crazy on a shopping cart, or the kind that glares at the brat a few feet away who's hacking up their lungs.

I will never ever strip my kid nearly naked in public. No, not even for a gravity-defying diarrhea blow out. I will never take blackmail pictures, use the television to distract them so I can actually *for the love of God* get something done, let them out of the house in mismatched ill-fitting clothes, post things online that have the potential to horrify them once they are old enough to feel things like embarrassment and shame, or let them cry instead of coddling their fake booboos. No no no! I will never be *that* kind of mom!

Clearly, I was smoking crack.

The biggest mistake anyone can make entering into the battlefield we call "parenthood" is thinking they have *any* damn idea of what it's going to be like. *My* biggest mistake was thinking there was a specific mold I had to fit into, a specific way I needed to feel or act or carry myself to truly be the mom I thought I *should* be. I shouldn't have thought anything. How much does *that* go against what everyone tells you? I wish someone would have sat my panicky ass down and told me to forget the stereotypical nonsense and just go with it. That no one's journey is the same; it can't be because it changes daily! Maybe even hourly! No two kids are exactly alike, so why in the hell would two parents have to be? As much as I said it, as many times as I swore it, as ridiculous as I know some of those things are to be doing or not doing or allowing. . . . Well, *that* kind of mom? Might just be me at times.

That kind of mom is sometimes a good mom, other times a great mom, and sometimes just an okay mom who dances along the line of "totally crazy maybe call the authorities" mom, but it's me, and I *am* a mom. That alone is pretty badass. I'm not sure why it took so long to convince me, I mean . . . I grew two humans *inside my body,* and then I gave birth to them—through my frickin' *vagina*! Even if we just so happen to poop on the table, this whole parent thing is nothing to be ashamed of. It's fucking awesome.

Why the hell was I so crazy for the first few years? I blame all the rainbows and butterfly bullshit being floated around about how easy and wonderful parenthood is. And TV! And video games! And the hole in the ozone! But mostly, I blame me.

Having children of our own isn't just useful in showing us what is truly important in life (or just how many times we're willing to wear a shirt before calling it "dirty" because we want to avoid doing the eleventh fucking load of laundry that week); it also shows you that you really *are* a superhero. I'm serious! We may not have pom poms, or have all of our shit together, and some days we may *start* the day with our barrel of patience completely empty, but in our own unique ways, we're all peppy, hand-standing, rah rah-ing, obnoxious cheerleaders. I even annoy *myself* sometimes.

I have a fucking coupon drawer, for God's sake.

My mom, the epitome of what I thought was the "cheerleader mom," was the single most embarrassingly crazy, outrageous, overbearing person I have ever known, and I'm proud to be just like her and nothing like her at the same time—even if it sucked really frickin' hard to prove her right time and time again. Tube socks were never necessary, and I don't have to join the PTA. *Parent* might be the title we hold, but it's more than just a job, more than just what you do. It becomes an integral part of who you are, and even though it changes you, *it* changes too. I'm gonna go all Mr. Rogers on you right now and tell you that parenthood is whatever the hell you want it to be.

I can't change the way other people think, or the way I think they think, but I can change how *I* think, and that's all I really needed to do. That, and to stop being so ridiculously dense and stubborn, but one thing at a time here, people!

I may not exactly always be proud of the lengths I will go to at times. It may even slightly embarrass me when I realize too much of my mom-ness is showing and I'll tuck that shit back in, but it's me, and probably you, too. Because we love our kids, and love can tend to be irrational, ridiculous, and completely insane. When it comes to taking care of our own, or making them happy, or even keeping ourselves sane enough to take care of them day in and day out, well, I guess that makes a little bit of batshit craziness in our blood okay.

Children, by nature, are horrible, wonderful, terrible, fantastic, evil, lovable, confusing, and infuriating miniature humans who will make their parents' lives feel whole while also driving them to the brink of insanity. Did they finally succeed in their evil mission to break me? Hell yes, they *absolutely* broke me, but in the best possible way. It feels like I've been through a war, and most of the time I have no earthly idea whether I've won or lost because, like a dumbass, the only thing I was fighting was myself. I've done things I never thought I'd do, said things I *swore* I'd never say, but what really showed me that I am a parent, a *mom*, through and through, and will never be the same? All of these sacrifices I have made for these kids; the privacy, the backwash floaty-filled drinks, the booger-free shirts, and the uninterrupted bowel movements . . . These don't feel like sacrifices at all. Except sleep; sleep was most definitely a sacrifice.

I think that's what people call "growing"—and that is one of the amazing benefits to bringing a tiny, needy, obnoxious, poop-filled human into your home.

Even though I've been broken and will finally accept and submit to the title of Parent, no matter how disgustingly booger-bubble-blowing sappy and sentimental I get, no matter how crazy overprotective helicoptering booboo kissing tooth fairy impersonating I become, I refuse to lose the ongoing battle between my ass, denim, and gravity. No matter how far I fall down this rabbit hole, I will still never *ever* wear mile-long camel toe causing mom jeans. That's a promise. Ask my kids—I am annoying about keeping those, *especially* when it comes to punishments.

I am a mom. There. I said it. I get it, I own it, I'm even proud of it now. But, while *you* can call me that, to my kids? It had *better* be Mommy.

ACKNOWLEDGEMENTS

To my children—for always being an inspiration, be it good or bad. You are both amazing, hilarious, annoying, stubborn, and wonderful humans. I can't wait to see what kind of havoc you wreak on the world.

To my husband—for never being one of the turds who questions why I didn't get a "real" job.

To my friends—who read draft after draft and never complained, listened to me bitch without judging, and talked me through it when my head felt like it was going to explode. You are the best there is.

To my dad—the strongest person I know. You might not get me, but you have been the rock of my life. The one who showed me how to laugh at adversity and ridiculous family nonsense. Without you, I would not be me.

To my agent, Maria Ribas—for believing in me when it was beginning to feel like no one else did. You are amazing, and you helped shape not only my book, but me as a writer. I couldn't have done this without you.

To my editor, Nicole Frail—for not cringing and running away at my overuse of run-on sentences and crazy punctuation, and for encouraging (and honing) my ridiculousness. Thank you!

And to my mom—for being obnoxiously right, all the time.